AMONGST THE VILLAGE MAGAZINE

Winter 2024 Issue

Powered by the
*Perinatal Resource Collaborative
A Division of HARLOT Co. &
Womb Light Energy LLC.*

For information about special discounts or bulk
purchases, please contact Sales at
prcvillage@gmail.com

Founder's Note

Birth is a journey for every woman, mother and family to explore on their own terms. This issue of Amongst the Village is to showcase the options and opportunities that exist within the birthing spectrum. Not to discredit other birthing stories, options or experiences. We encourage everyone to do their own independent research and choose the option that fits your needs the best.

Nicole Harlet

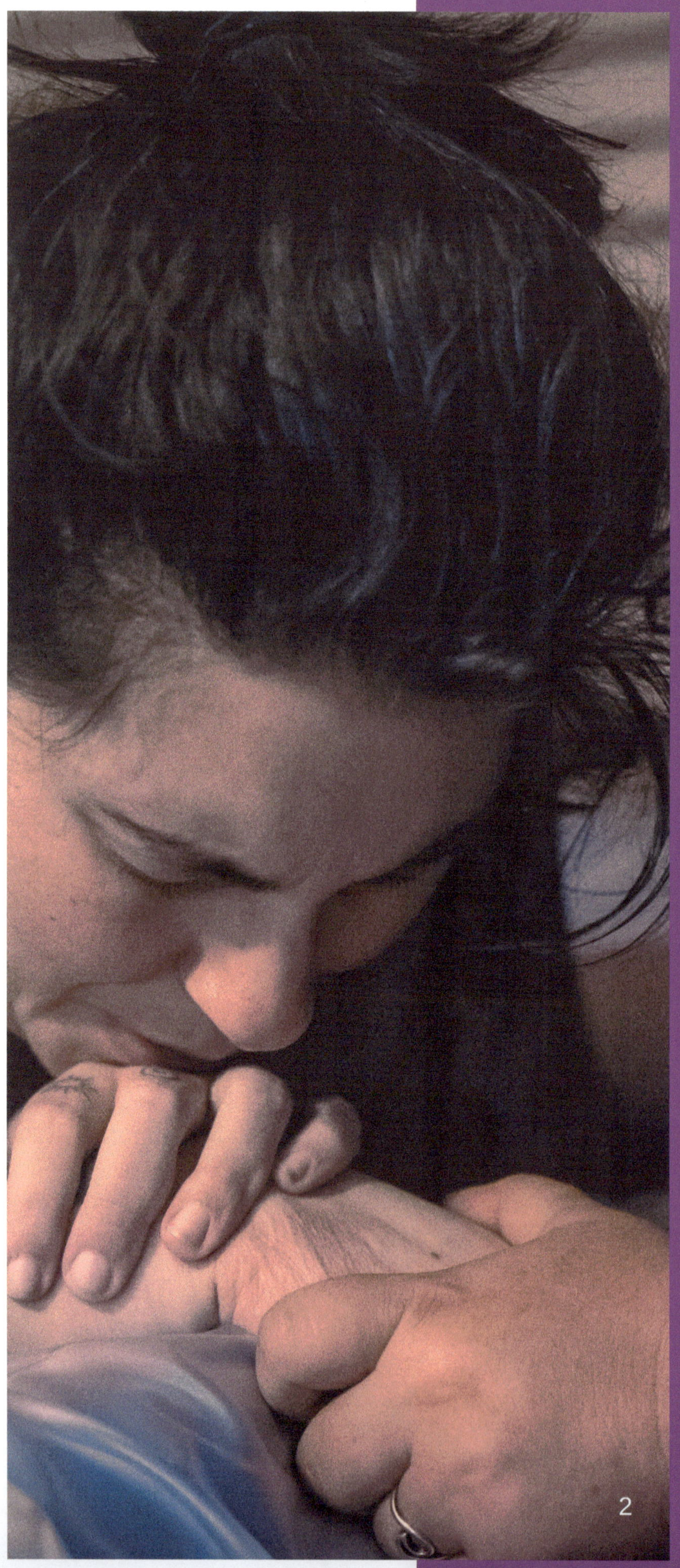

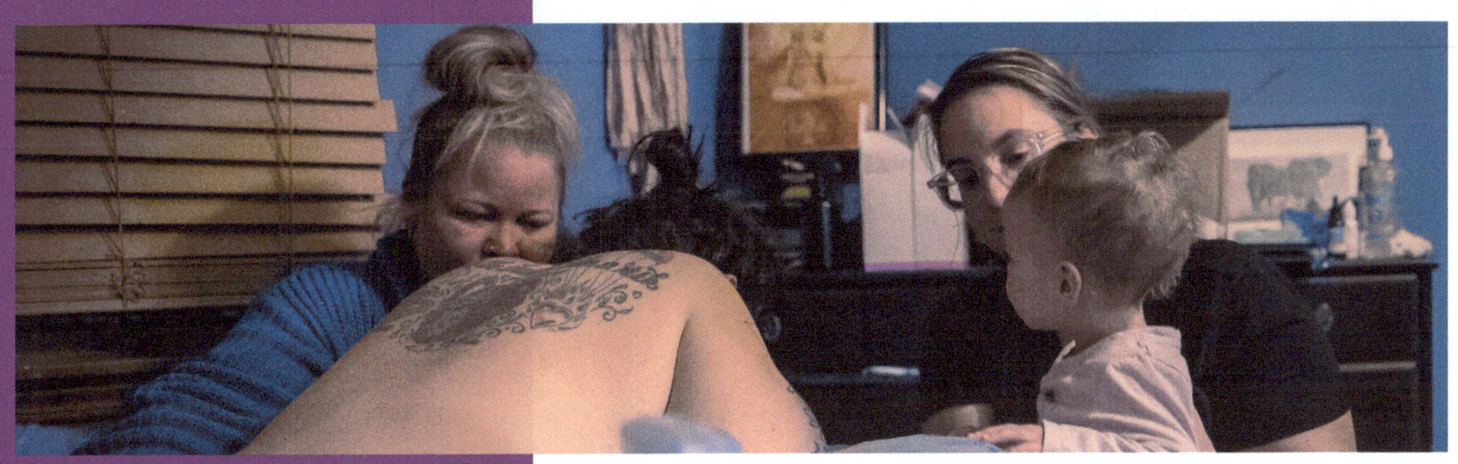

A PEEK AT WHAT'S WITHIN

& MORE

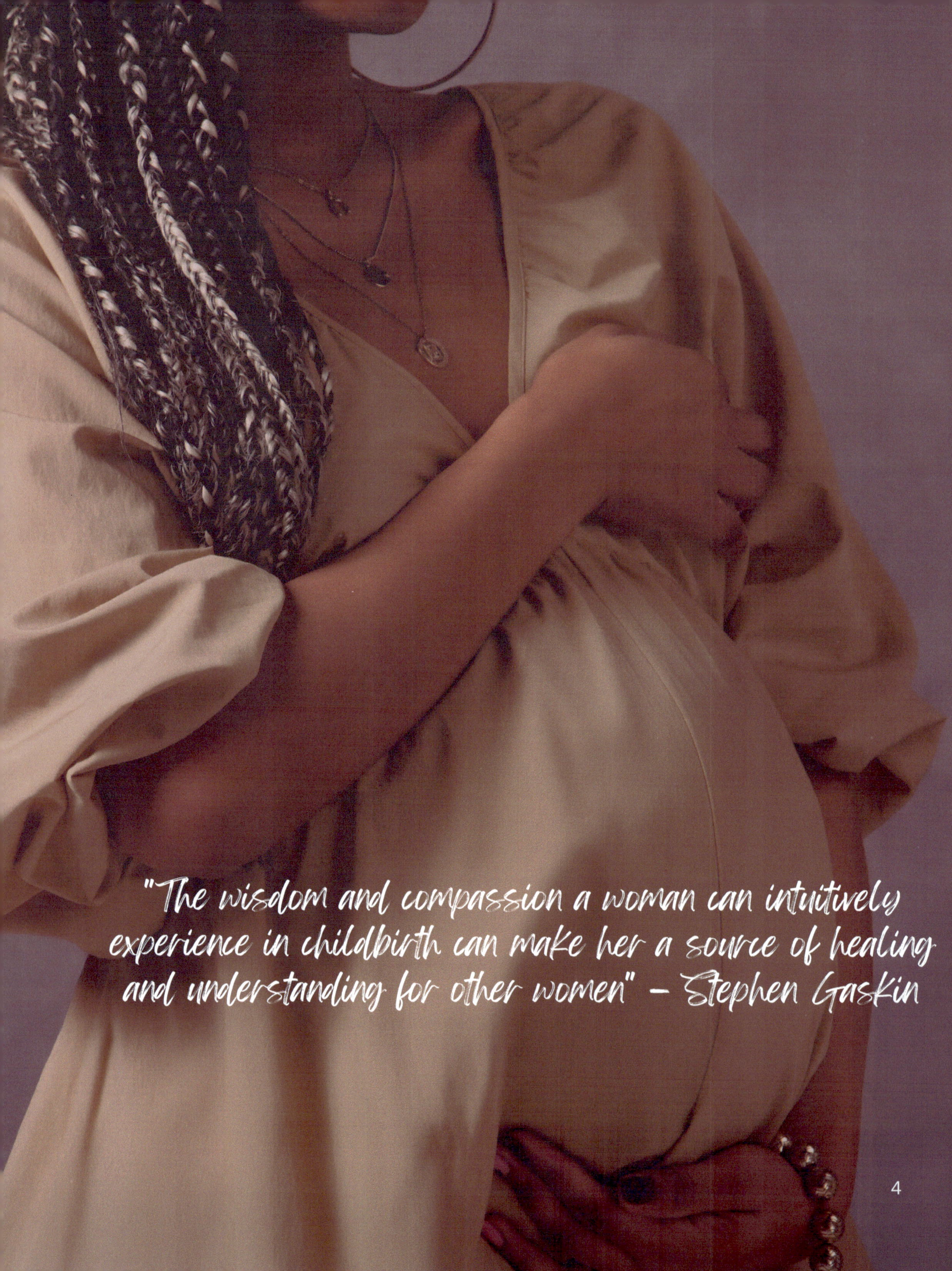
"The wisdom and compassion a woman can intuitively experience in childbirth can make her a source of healing and understanding for other women" - Stephen Gaskin

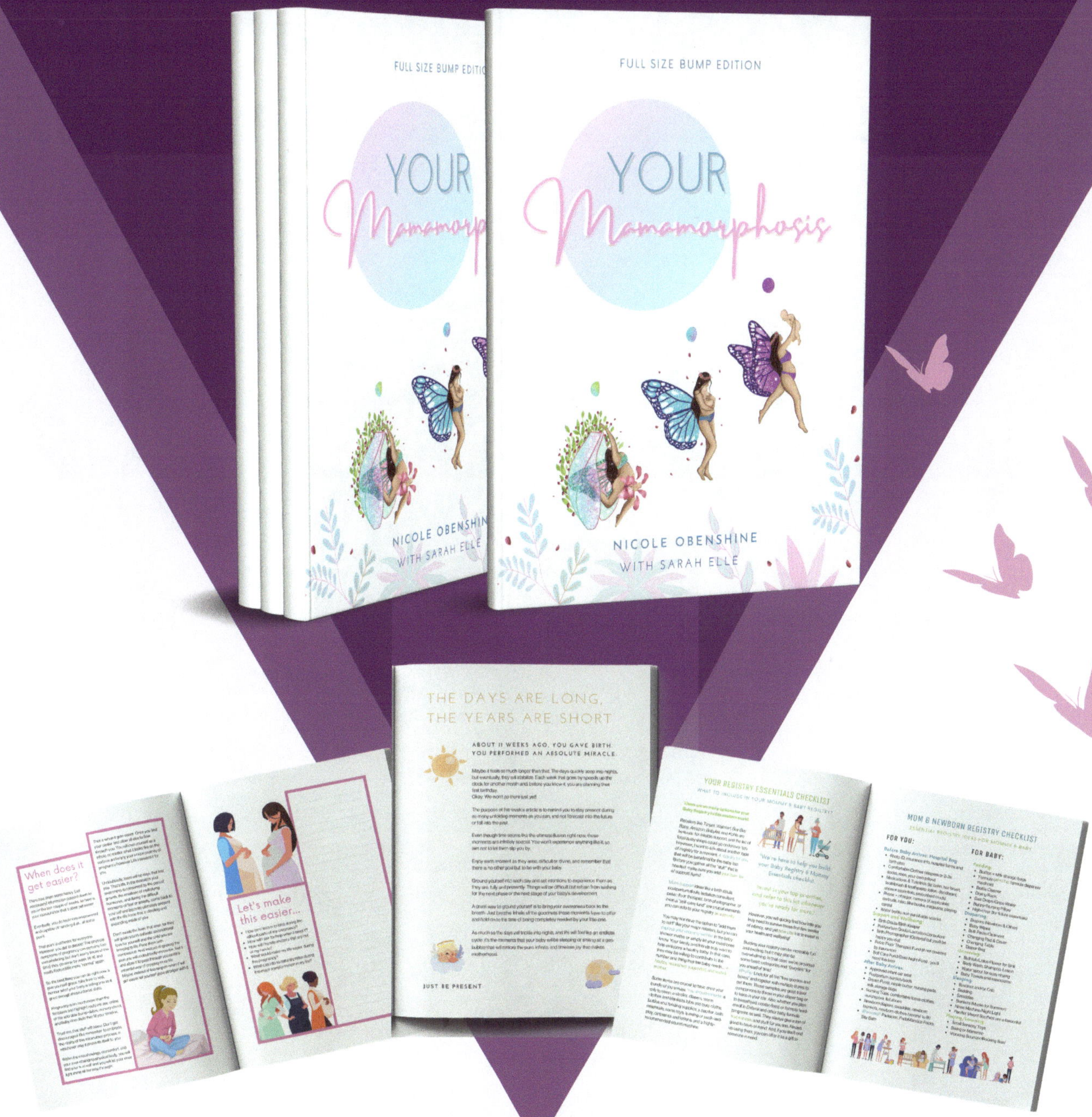

Get access to articles for all four trimesters, supportive journal prompts, birth and postpartum plan templates, a space for your birth story, an affirmation poster, and real experiences and stories from moms. This tangible resource for your journey is available for *only $10.*

FLOWCODE
PRIVACY.FLOWCODE.COM

SCAN QR CODE TO PURCHASE

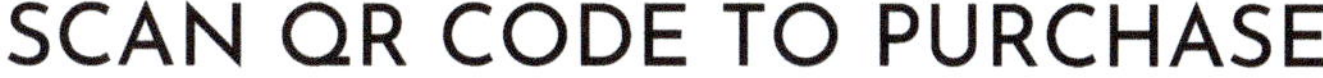

Home is Where Birth Is

By Sarah Zadoyko-Bartee

I was twenty-five years old and expecting my first child with limited knowledge on "what's next". As with most future moms, I made my first appointment with my OBGYN, and it was an experience I shall never forget. From sitting in the cold waiting room, being interrogated with what felt to be a million questions, the lack of care for my responses, and the overall uncomfortable feeling. Although my feelings were unsettling, I knew no other path towards motherhood, I was not a "rule breaker" or someone who pushes against society at that time. After only a 15-minute appointment, I left the office with my next appointment scheduled four weeks out.

The stomach flu left me bedridden for several days where Netflix and documentaries kept me company. One came across as recommended called "The Business of Being Born" and with excitement, I watched. This documentary opened my eyes to exactly what the title entails – the business of childbirth. I knew I did not want to be a part of that machine. I did not want to have a baby in the hospital. Now, with my mind racing, I started conducting intense research on my options. Midwifery held my interest from first look as the process seems more intimate and inclusive rather than a model of business.

My first appointment with SoulShine Midwifery, I felt relieved and wholeheartedly knew that homebirth was the path for my family. The appointment left me feeling in control, feeling informed, feeling valued, and feeling cared for. Throughout the process of my child's birth, this did not change once. The care and attention were priceless. The ability to give birth in my home kept stress levels minimal. Having the people of my choosing present, meant the world to me.

The time came for my first child's birth, and it was a doozy with 23 hours and 58 minutes of labor. In retrospect, it was delightful compared to the horror stories I would later hear from friends and witness as a doula. I was not rushed, I was not confined to a bed, I was not pressured to take an epidural, and I was not poked or prodded in any way. I was beyond thankful that I retained my freedom to move, eat, sleep, walk, and do anything I wanted to do. After laboring in a birth tub, I felt the urge to bear down. I removed myself from the tub and sat on the toilet for a few minutes, had a few contractions, and a crest of my baby's head was there. My midwife and husband helped me back to the warm tub where a few moments later my husband helped catch our baby and announced the gender – girl. It was an unforgettable moment. My first daughter was a healthy 8 pounds, 9 ounces.

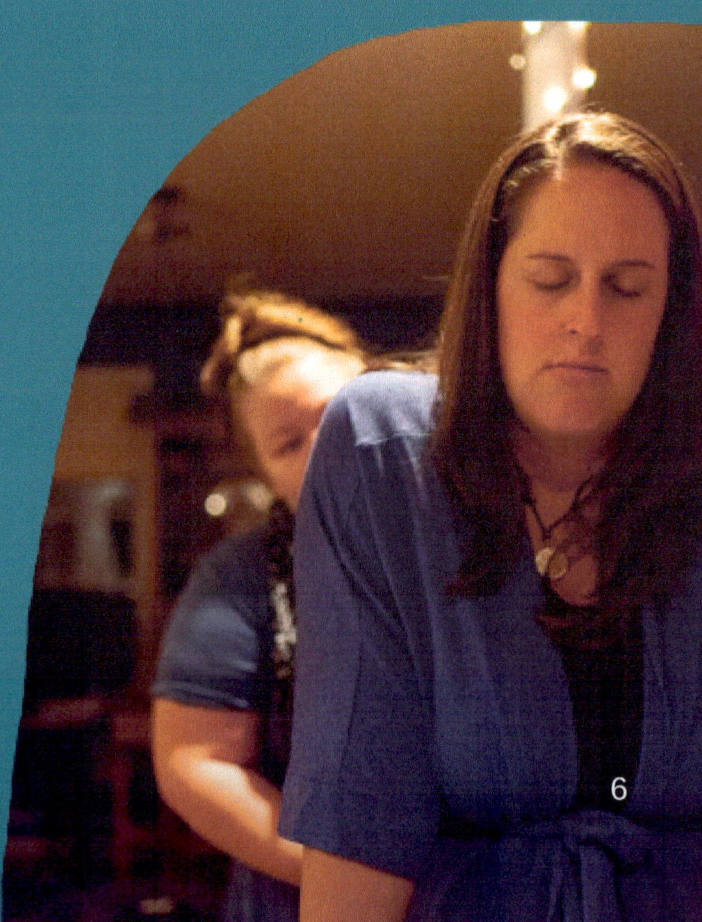

Shortly after our daughter was born, I had to get out of the water because my placenta was not coming out and it is difficult to tell how much you are bleeding in water. We moved to my bedroom where I remained in a complete oxytocin bubble and in pure bliss. There was never a concern from me that things were out of control, or regret that I was not in the hospital. The midwife kept a keen eye on me the whole night and even when I lost consciousness momentarily, she was prepared. My husband remained calm and told me the situation was not cause for worry as he saw the professional in the midwife. Ultimately, my placenta was delivered and the bleeding stopped. I had lost more blood than was desired but, recovered quickly, and my midwife stayed the night to ensure my health and welfare.

Flash forward nearly two years and I would be preparing to give birth again. This time I was able to have discussions with my midwife and balance the likelihood of a retained placenta and bleeding once again. Needless to say, my confidence in her skills and abilities remained high as I chose to once again have a home birth. This labor was completely different and lasted only 2 hours. This little boy was determined to join us in this world so quickly we never had time to prepare the tub. Everything was fast paced and when the bleeding came, we had a plan. The paramedics were on standby and when we thought we might use them, the placenta detached, and bleeding stopped. Once again, a prepared environment leading to a worry-free experience. My first son was a whopping 10 pounds, 2 ounces.

Six months later I discovered I was pregnant once again and would be blessed with a fourth baby which I assumed would go similar to my third. One could not be more wrong. The labor and delivery were absolutely flawless and this time, I decided to catch the baby – my baby girl. I was on cloud nine; however, my midwife noticed the water getting darker and told me to get out of the water. This girl was 11 pounds, 12 ounces and the placenta did not want to detach. My midwife performed her role flawlessly but despite all her efforts a transfer to the hospital was needed.

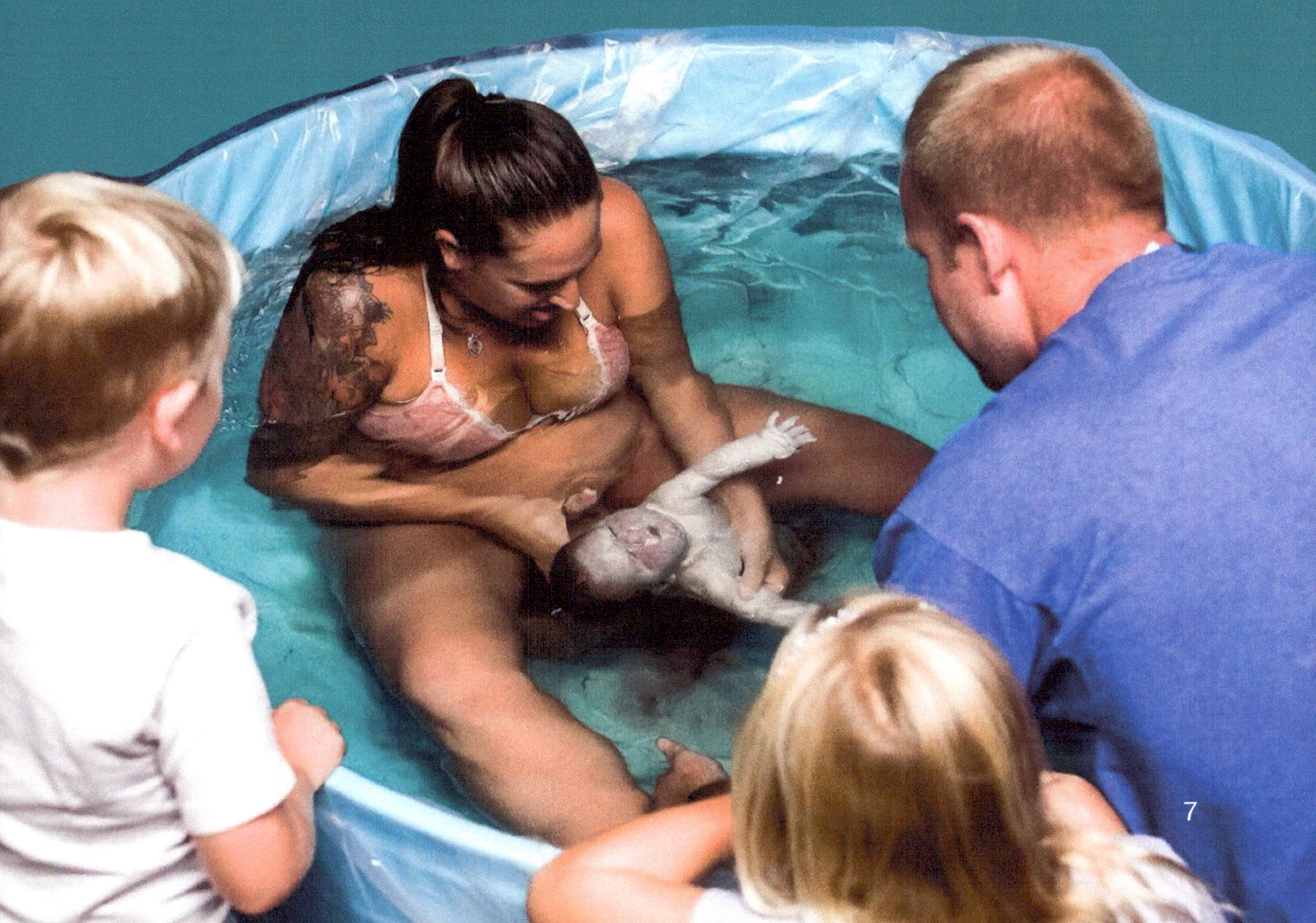

Arrival at the hospital was interesting to say the least. It was 2020 and the COVID-19 pandemic was in full throttle. Although actively bleeding and having no symptoms of being ill, it was question after question about who I have been in contact with, insurance verification, and requirements to get swabbed for COVID. The OBGYN on call attempted to do a manual extraction (pull out) my placenta to no success. She decided I would need to be taken to the operating room for surgical removal. The hospital staff began to prepare me for surgery and the anesthesiologist came to ask me more questions and shamed me for choosing a homebirth. I could feel the blood pooling under my bottom and they were more concerned COVID and questioning my choices than caring for the condition I was there for. It wasn't until my blood pressure dropped to dangerous levels that they rushed me back to the OR.

The last thing I remembered hearing was that they couldn't find any blood for me. Luckily once placed under anesthesia, my placenta detached without intervention and my bleeding stopped immediately. No surgery occurred. The hospital was unable to get blood for me until I had been back in my room for about thirty minutes. At each step of this hospital journey, I felt policy triumphed over my health and welfare. I was told my baby could not join me in the hospital because she wasn't born there. That was the straw that broke me. I signed an AMA statement and went home to my loving family.

Despite all I went through with my last child, if I were to have another baby, home birth would be the only path for me. After my first child I decided that I wanted to be involved in helping women become mothers through birth work. I became a birth and postpartum doula, lactation consultant, placenta encapsulater and birth photographer. I have worked with mothers taking care of them before, during and after childbirth for ten years now. You can imagine that I have heard and also witnessed just about all that can go right and wrong in the journey to meeting your baby both in and out of the hospital. I encourage each mother-to-be and family to perform research, take opinions, and get involved in your own care. You only get to meet your baby for the first time once. That experience can be cold and business oriented placing policy above all else or it can be personal, supported and empowering where you get to take back control of what your body was designed to do as a woman. (Without algorithms, community standards, or sensitive content warnings getting in your way!)

The benefits and opportunities to contribute are growing and limitless. The mission is to be the village for the villagers and to fill the gaps for one another, supporting the global collective of those we serve.

If you are an expecting or new mom reading this, please share the name Perinatal Resource Collaborative with anyone who supports you during your perinatal period so they can also be supported and have opportunities to share their stories and expertise in various ways.

Together, we thrive and rise—it is a village circle.

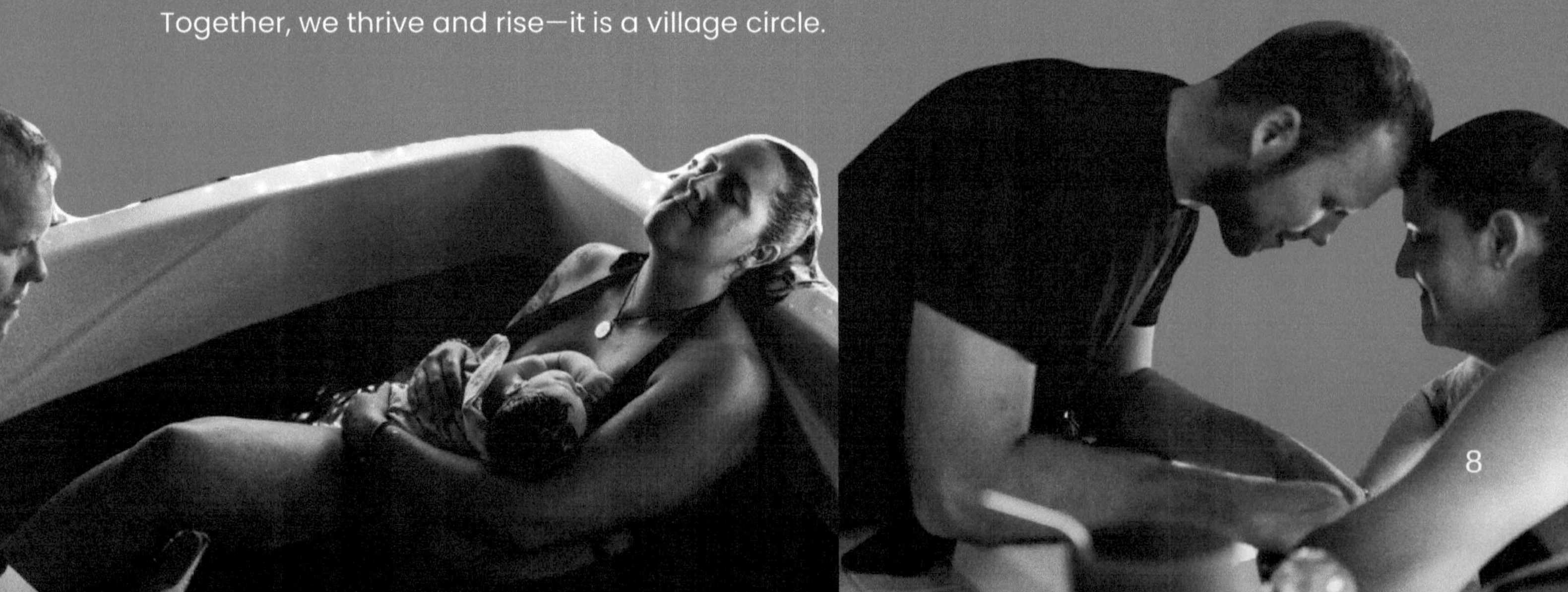

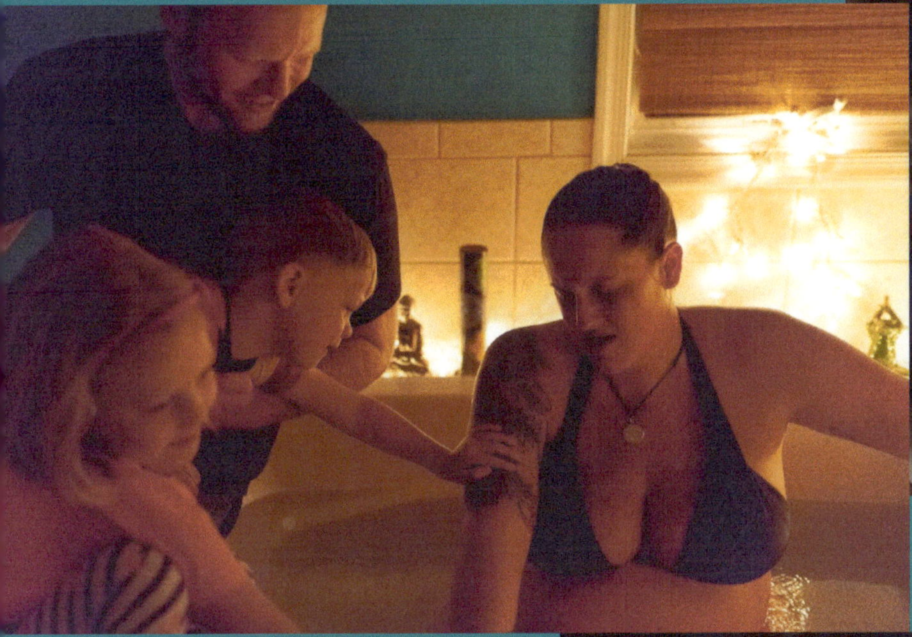

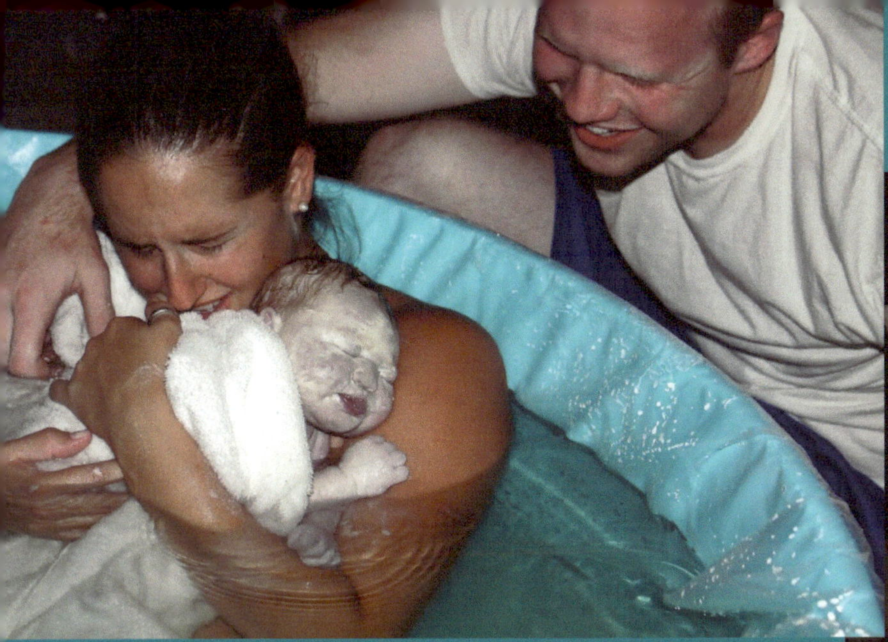

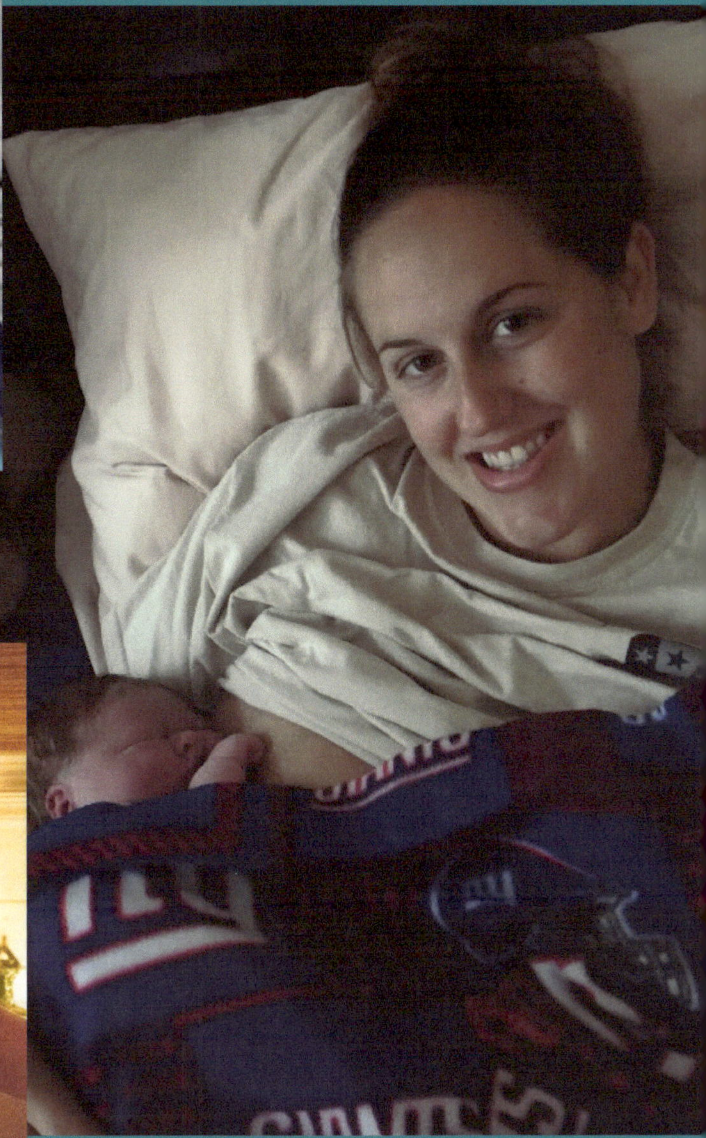

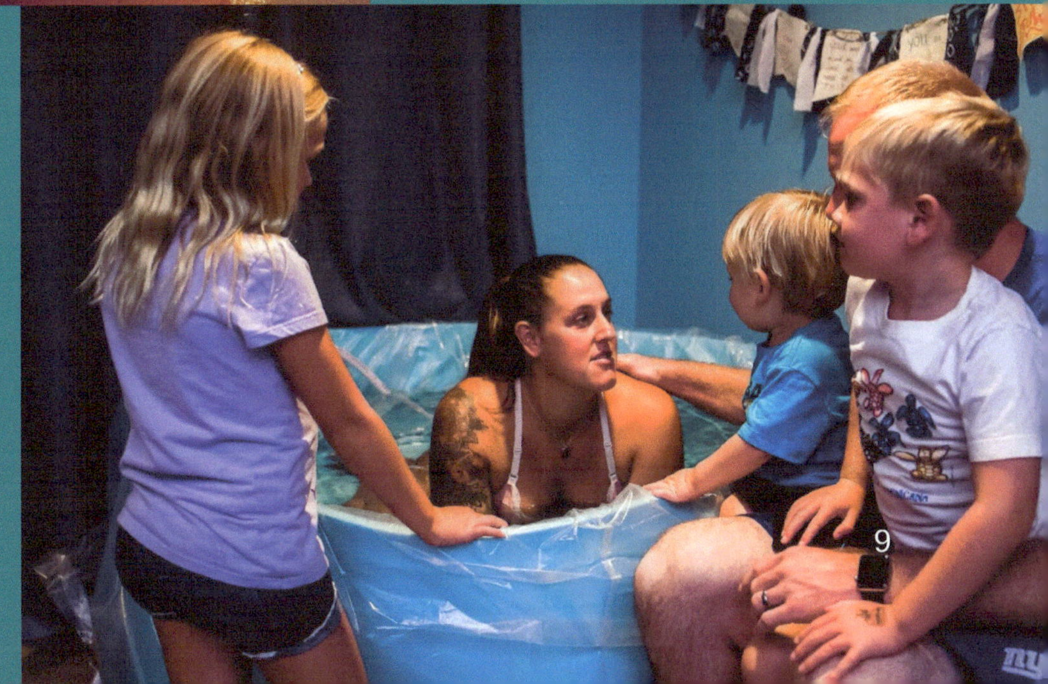

Sarah Zadoyko-Bartee
The Mamma Warrior USA
Birth Photographer, Full
Spectrum Doula, CLC,
Placenta Encapsulator
New Jersey Based

Find her online
@themammawarrior

birth**ify**.

Your Digital Doula From Bump to Baby

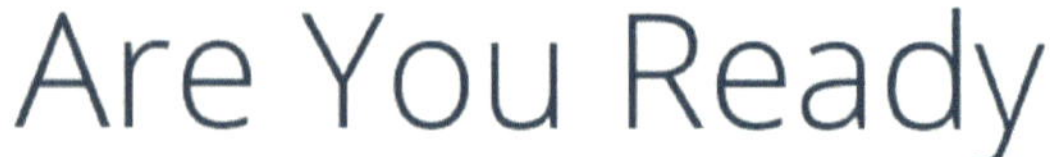

Are You Ready

For a Smoother Birth and Postpartum Experience?

Finally, the Support Every New Parent Has Always Needed

Scan Me

- **Full-spectrum doula care for pregnancy, birth, postpartum, and newborn care**

- **Available 24/7 through messaging and virtual coaching**

- **More affordable than traditional doula services**

- **Get answers to questions you didn't know to ask**

www.birthify.net

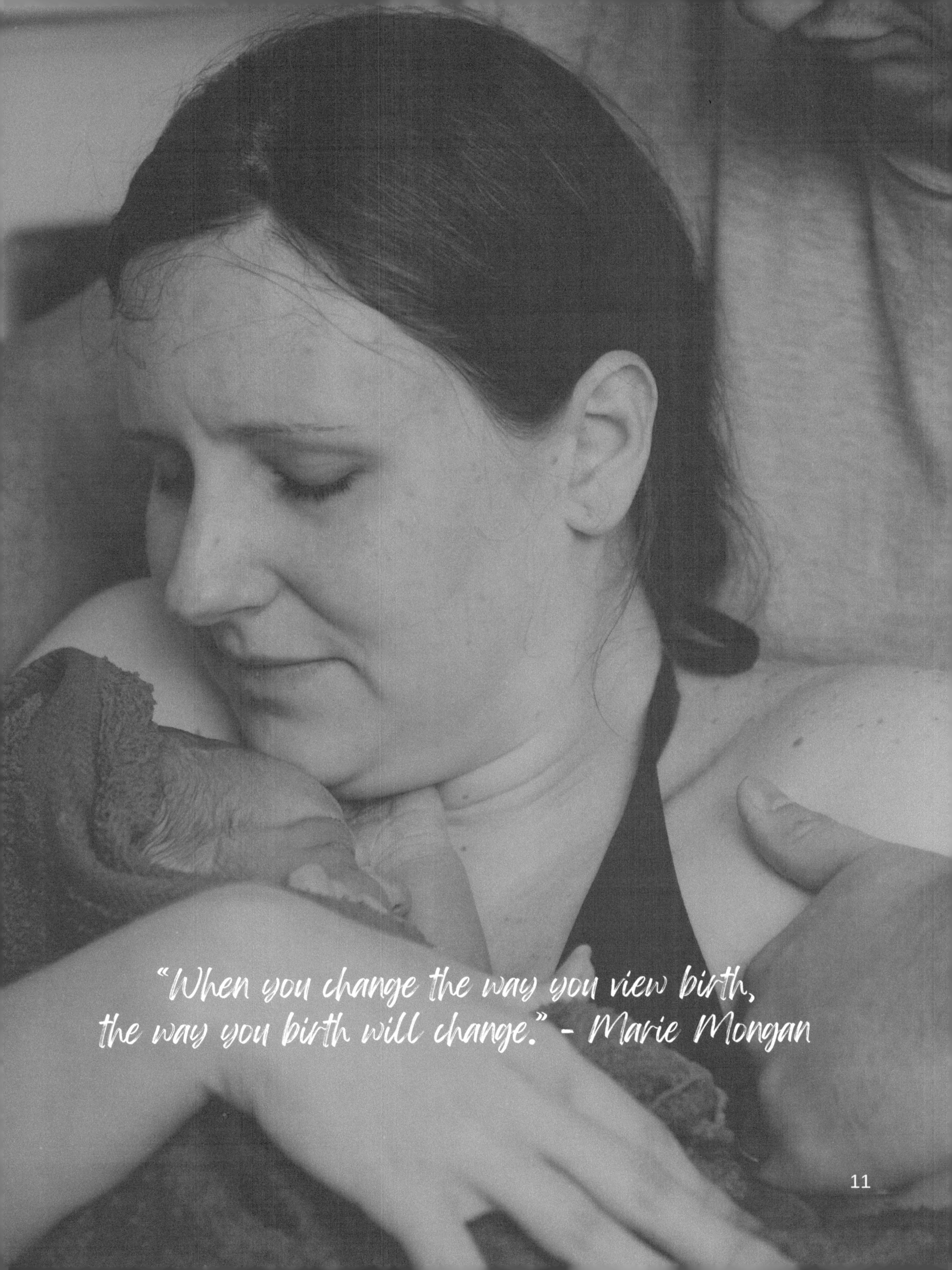

"When you change the way you view birth,
the way you birth will change." - Marie Mongan

HOMEBIRTH STORIES

Summary of the Submissions:

Of the 10+ Submissions, about half were within the water and half were out of water. Additionally, we had about 95% Assisted with a Midwife and 5% Unassisted. All had support teams including a spouse/partner, other family members, existing children and doulas.

ALL of them said they would do it again. On the next page you will see some snippets from their submissions and quotes from their stories.

Thank you to Hollie F., Karen K., Abbie M., Emerald W., Rachael N., Sara L., Danielle T., Nichole F., Marie R., Chrissy K. and the others who submitted.

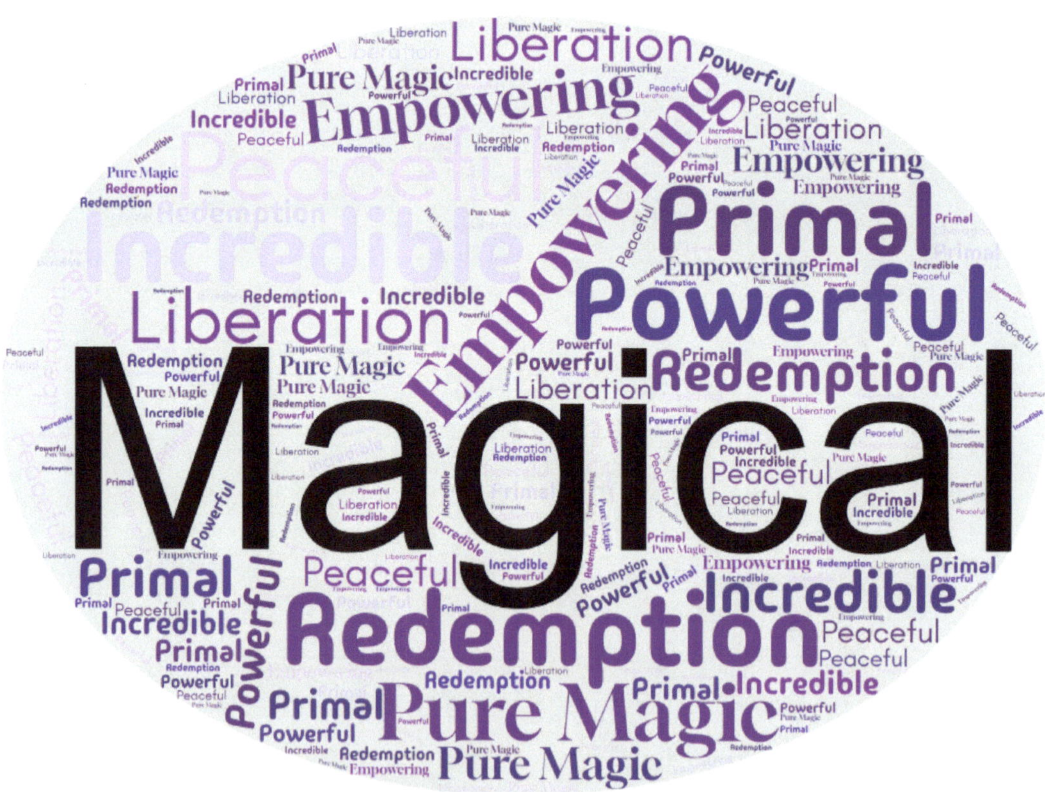

Choosing a homebirth was one of the most transformative decisions I have ever made. Now, looking back, I only wish I'd chosen this path from the start, because every moment of my homebirth felt like pure magic. Being in the water felt unlike anything I had ever experienced. I had the freedom to move, to feel the weightlessness and the natural relief it offered. It was as if the water itself was guiding me through the final stages of labor, bringing my body and mind into a state of profound calm. There were no cords, no tubes, just me, my breath, and the soothing waters as I prepared to meet my baby. With my eyes closed, I silently breathed him out, moving entirely with the rhythms of my body. The midwife's soft voice broke through my focus,There is his head. And just seconds later, he was in my arms, his tiny body warm against mine. That moment was the most real, the most natural thing I have ever done.

My homebirth brought me a peace and joy I had never felt before. It was an experience filled with intimacy, beauty, and strength a memory I will hold close for the rest of my life. I am grateful beyond words for the chance to bring my baby into the world, right where we both belonged.

I had an amazing midwife who trusted my body 100% I carried 44w 1d before going into labor. I labored for 6 hours after my water broke. I moved from my bed to the shower a lot to relieve back pain. When it was time to push I was in my bed. Fetal ejection reflex was strongly taking over and my body was working beautifully to push my baby out. Her shoulders got stuck (shoulder dystocia) but my midwife kept calm. Which kept me and my husband calm. We worked together to get her out. I pushed for about 2 minutes and then she was in my arms! This was my 4th baby and the first time I got to hold my baby after delivery. My first two were C-sections, and my 3rd was a hospital vbac. I felt so much relief and redemption during the whole experience. After an hour of holding her skin to skin and nursing, she was weighed up. She was 11lbs!!!!!! I had no tearing at all. My body, and baby worked well together to deliver her big beautiful self. When I surrendered everything it all clicked into place! I'd do it 100 times more if I could. It was the most powerful, and uplifting experience of my life!

Quiet and serene. In bedroom with dim lights and low music. In and out of the tub. Most incredible experience of my life. Slow, but controlled and peaceful.

I had the perfect first time mom homebirth! I wanted to share because reading other peoples was so inspiring to me. I'm a big nerdy scientist, so I read all the stats before I decided this was the birth for me, and I still had in my head the high probability of hospital transfer. I'd had a very healthy uncomplicated pregnancy, but my blood pressure was starting to rise at 39 weeks, so I wanted baby to come sooner rather than later. The midwives were measuring baby's heart rate after contractions and reminding me to take deep slow breaths to re-oxygenate. Finally I started to feel that ring of fire thing - which wasn't any more painful than any other part of the process, but also not so much a relief as a good guide for where to push. I got his head out a few contractions later, and then his body was stuck until the next contraction - the shoulders were the most painful part! But then he was there on my chest and a few seconds later, crying and squirming and making all the cutest sounds I've ever heard in my life.

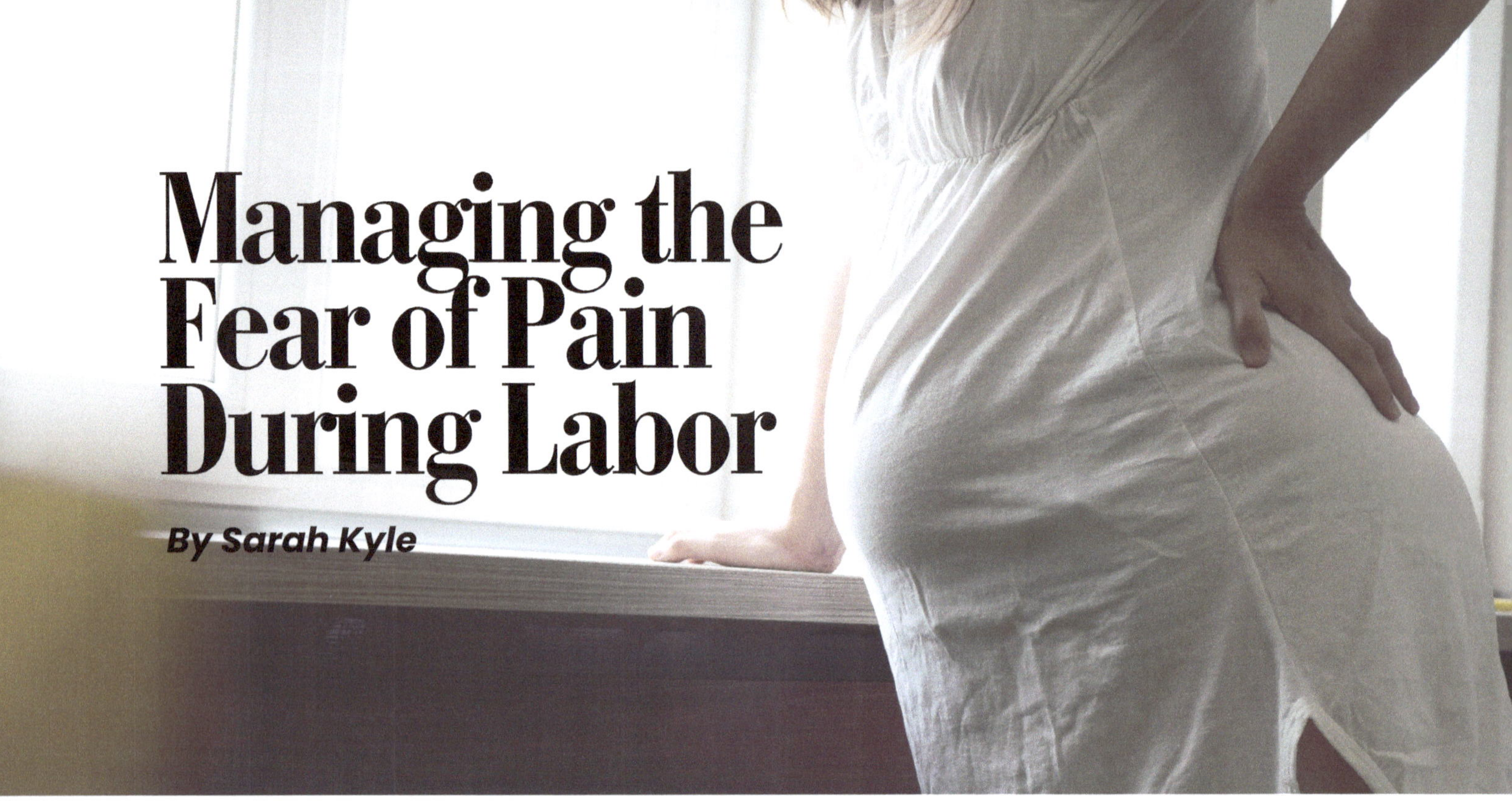

Managing the Fear of Pain During Labor

By Sarah Kyle

Congratulations Mama! You are officially reaching a stage in your pregnancy journey where you are wanting to learn more about pain management! Yes that's right pain management, for those who said their birth wasn't painful are one of five things. They have a high pain tolerance, psyche was in the right place creating a serine moment of a hormone infused birth, medicated with a nerve blocker such as an epidural, unfortunately lied to you, or successfully managed their labor with comfort techniques. If you're reading this, you are probably curious on what type of pain management is available to you?

There are 2 categories: natural pain relief and medical pain relief (analgesics). Now, not all techniques of pain management have the same outcome for everybody. Some simply can breathe their pains away while others need a little more umph. Today we will discuss natural pain relief as well as the possibility of pain relief a Midwife may administer during a home birth.

"Pain is a natural part of labor, but it doesn't have to control you. By understanding your options and utilizing effective comfort techniques, you can actively manage your pain and have a positive birth experience." Penny Simkin[1]

First, I want to state that your psyche plays a major role during your birth. If you have any fear or doubt about your labor, or what things will be like post natal, this can affect your birth. Having fear, anxiety or being uncomfortable can allow the hormone adrenaline to cut off oxytocin, the hormone used to induce labor. Oxytocin is the birth hormone, healing hormone as well as the hormone that encourages milk let down. Having items around you during your labor that encourages oxytocin release can assist your labor.

Think of your 5 senses; sight, smell, taste, touch and hear. Make a list of items within your 5 senses that you like; a massage anywhere on your body, the smell of roses or vanilla, the taste of a fresh baked cookie, pineapple juice or a savory treat. Dimming the lights, a warm bath, and your favorite essential oil in your diffuser or candle burning in the background can all comfort you during labor and encourage oxytocin release. Using a comb during your contractions, hot or cold compress, or even taking a walk outside can encourage a more peaceful labor. Having a Doula (non-medical professional) at your birth can benefit you as they can encourage you to do labor positions to open your hips, help with breathing techniques, as well as assist you or help your partner with comfort techniques. As well as, assist with Miles circuit techniques and hypnobirthing as comfort measures.

Doulas provide much needed emotional support for you and your partner as you endure the marathon of birth together. Birth is painful, there's no doubt about that! However, the comfort techniques you use can significantly decrease the pain receptors from taking precedence. Take the time now to watch videos, find a Doula who matches your needs of support, a Midwife that accepts your wishes, and learn how to provide comfort for yourself during labor.

Secondly, if you decide to pursue your home birth you will need a Midwife (medical professional) to assist in delivering your baby Earth side. Your Midwife can be as hands on or off as you wish, they will support you with labor positions, checking your and babies heart rate, if desired, and perform cervical checks and many more tasks. In saying that, there are an abundance of great midwives out there, however there are different types of Midwives (CPM, LM, DEM, CNM) each license allows that midwife to only perform what the state allows.

Each state will have regulations on what a Midwife can give their patient medically outside of the hospital setting. Historically, Midwives would give an opioid such as pethidine, however that is not used in the states anymore. I have heard of Midwives who use medicinal herbs to create the same effects as some of the medications the hospital would give. I would recommend speaking to your Midwife or during your interviews ask what they can perform for pain relief during your homebirth.

You can ask about the TENS unit, Healy, drugs, interthecal, narcotics, as well as herbal supplements they can use or recommend during your birth. Never be afraid to ask about what is available to you. Never let your pain turn into suffering, just because you wanted an "unmedicated" birth. There are so many options for pain relief, comfort measures and distractions that can give you the relief you desire. Remember this is *your* birth, ask questions, hire a Doula who can help educate and support you, find a Midwife that suits your needs. You have a right to your birth, your body and your experiences. However, remember not all births follow a certain plan, things can change in an instant, mentally prepare yourself, get your support team planned out and write down your list of 5 senses items you want present at your birth. Congratulations Mama, on taking the next big step of learning about pain management, you got this!

"Confident Mamas make informed decisions" ~ Sarah Kyle, Doula.

[1]Simkin, P. (2018). Birth Partner 5th Edition: A Complete Guide to Childbirth for Dads, Partners, Doulas, and All Other Labor Companions. Harvard Common Press.

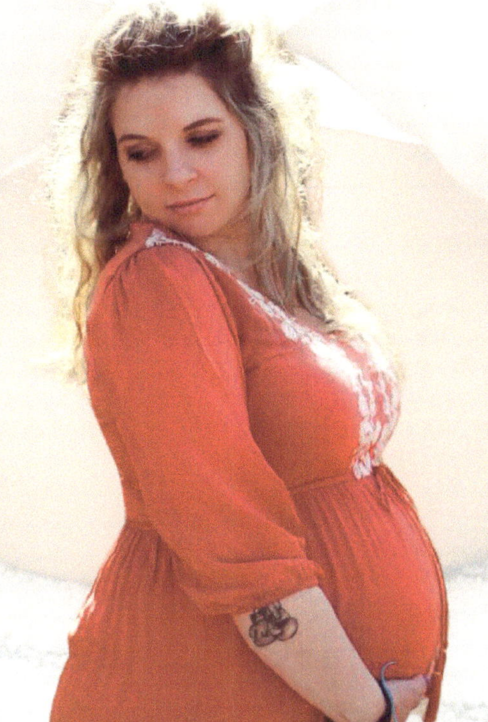

Sarah Kyle
Confident Mamas Doula
CLD, CISE
Based in Oklahoma
Find her online at @confident_mamas or
on Facebook at Confident Mamas

www.confidentmamasdoula.com

Exploring Home Births: A Journey Back to Nature with Modern Insights

By Debi Tracy

In recent years, the desire for a more personalized and intimate birthing experience has led many families to consider home births. This choice, rooted in tradition yet informed by contemporary healthcare practices, offers an empowering journey for expectant parents. By focusing on the roles of midwives, the importance of support teams, dispelling prevalent myths, and setting up a nurturing birth space, families can embrace a home birth with confidence and joy.

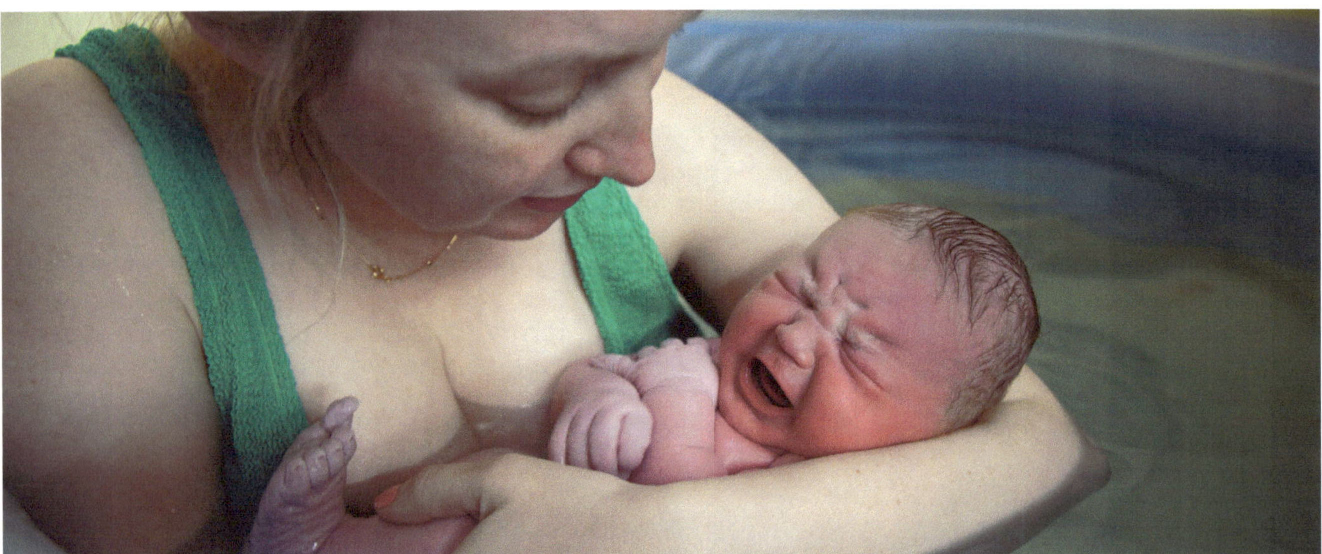

Welcoming Life: A Story of Serenely Empowered Birth

The decision to bring my second baby into the world at home was fueled by a deep desire for a natural and fulfilling birthing experience after teaching HypnoBirthing® for three years. Under the stars of a September night, our home transformed into a sanctuary of warmth and support, embodying the essence of home birth. Our experience with Gaia Midwifery, as a dedicated support team, illuminated the profound possibilities that home births present. Central to this experience was our daughter Mila, who had been welcomed four years earlier at Elizabeth Seton Birth Center in NYC with HypnoBirthing®. Her genuine curiosity and joy added an irreplaceable layer of love and anticipation.

The Roles of Midwives and Birth Teams

Midwives are the cornerstone of ensuring safety, comfort, and support during a home birth. Their expertise not only encompasses prenatal care and labor management but also includes emotional reassurance and guidance. As we welcomed our baby, our midwives became trusted partners, and their knowledge anchored us through the beautiful chaos of childbirth. Anna Westley, our doula, was a beacon of calm, guiding me through each contraction and surge.

Hiring a birth team enhances the home birth experience by providing continuous physical and emotional support. Their presence can alleviate anxiety and help you and your family remain focused on the labor process. For this birth, our friends and family, including Mila, formed a network of love and strength, each member playing a unique role in his arrival.

Considering Unassisted Births

Some families may explore unassisted home births, drawn by the desire for minimal intervention. However, it is vital to balance these desires with considerations of safety. For us, choosing to have professional support allowed for a seamless transition should complications have arisen, granting peace of mind during this birth. Each family's comfort with this decision, guided by consultation with healthcare professionals, is crucial to a successful outcome.

Debunking Myths About Home Births

Home births are often shrouded in misconceptions, ranging from concerns about safety to the availability of emergency care. However, current studies indicate that home births are equally as safe as hospital births for low-risk pregnancies when overseen by skilled practitioners. Our experience with this birth mirrored this truth; the arrival was both safe and natural, supported by an expert team. Another common myth is the belief that home births lack the means to handle emergencies. Yet, well-prepared birth teams are *trained* to anticipate and manage such situations, facilitating quick hospital transfers if needed.

Creating the Ideal Birth Space

The atmosphere of a home birth is deeply personal, fostering an environment that allows for movement, comfort, and privacy. For this birth, we took great care in creating a warm, welcoming space, complete with a birthing tub that provided relief and respite. Mila's presence brought light and joy, as she moved about with excitement at the prospect of meeting her new sibling. Lights were dimmed to create a serene backdrop, while comforting scents and gentle music infused our surroundings with peace. Essential supplies such as birthing pools, bedding, and medical supplies were also prepared, ensuring that our space was not just personal but also practical. Knowing that our baby would be welcomed into a safe environment, physically and emotionally, was a profound part of our preparation.

Embracing Traditional Postpartum Recovery

Following the birth, our home became a cocoon of rest and recovery. Traditional practices emphasize rest and bonding, allowing new mothers the time and space to heal naturally. The postpartum period is a time to cherish skin-to-skin contact and to gently nurture the bond with your newborn. Mila, who had waited patiently, embraced her new sibling with the joy of a newfound friend, announcing she had a brother with boundless excitement.

Our support network, who had lovingly assisted during the birth, continued to care for household duties, allowing us to focus solely on our son and each other. Embracing traditional postpartum recovery enhanced my healing, providing the emotional and physical support necessary for navigating early motherhood once again. Our family's teamwork extended beyond labor, fostering a nurturing environment in which to begin our life with our boy.

Celebrating a Personal Birth Journey

Home births offer a uniquely personalized entry into parenthood, blending the sanctity of tradition with the assurance of modern medical practices. Our experience, enriched by Mila's enthusiasm and involvement, underscored the strength and beauty inherent in this choice, affirming our belief in natural processes and the efficacy of a prepared support team. For those considering a home birth, the journey promises to be an enriching chapter in your family's story, defined by resilience, love, and the unfurling beauty of new life.

As a lasting testament to her role in this journey, Mila chose the name Lukas instead of Luke for her brother. She wanted his name to resonate with her own, giving it two syllables like hers, ensuring a harmonious bond through their names that reflected the closeness they share. This thoughtful gesture added yet another layer of love and individuality to Lukas' welcome, highlighting the deep bond already forming between siblings—a bond that continues to thrive almost two decades later.

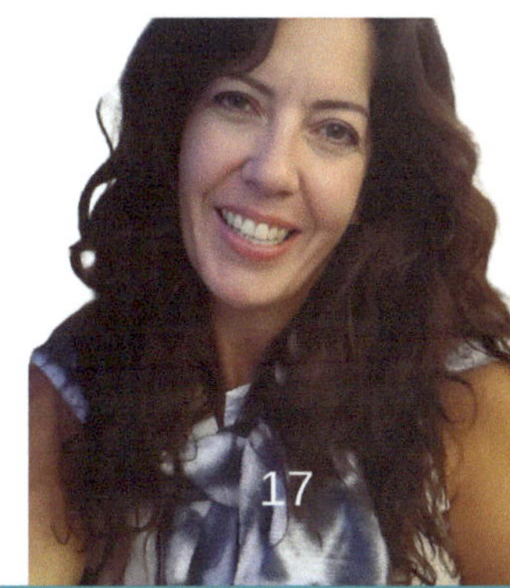

Debi Tracy
HYP MAMAS HUB
CHBCE, CH, CHBFS, E-RYT, RPYT,
CYBMI, CD, CMT
Find her on social media
@hyp_mamas_hub
Based in Long Island NY
Virtual Services too

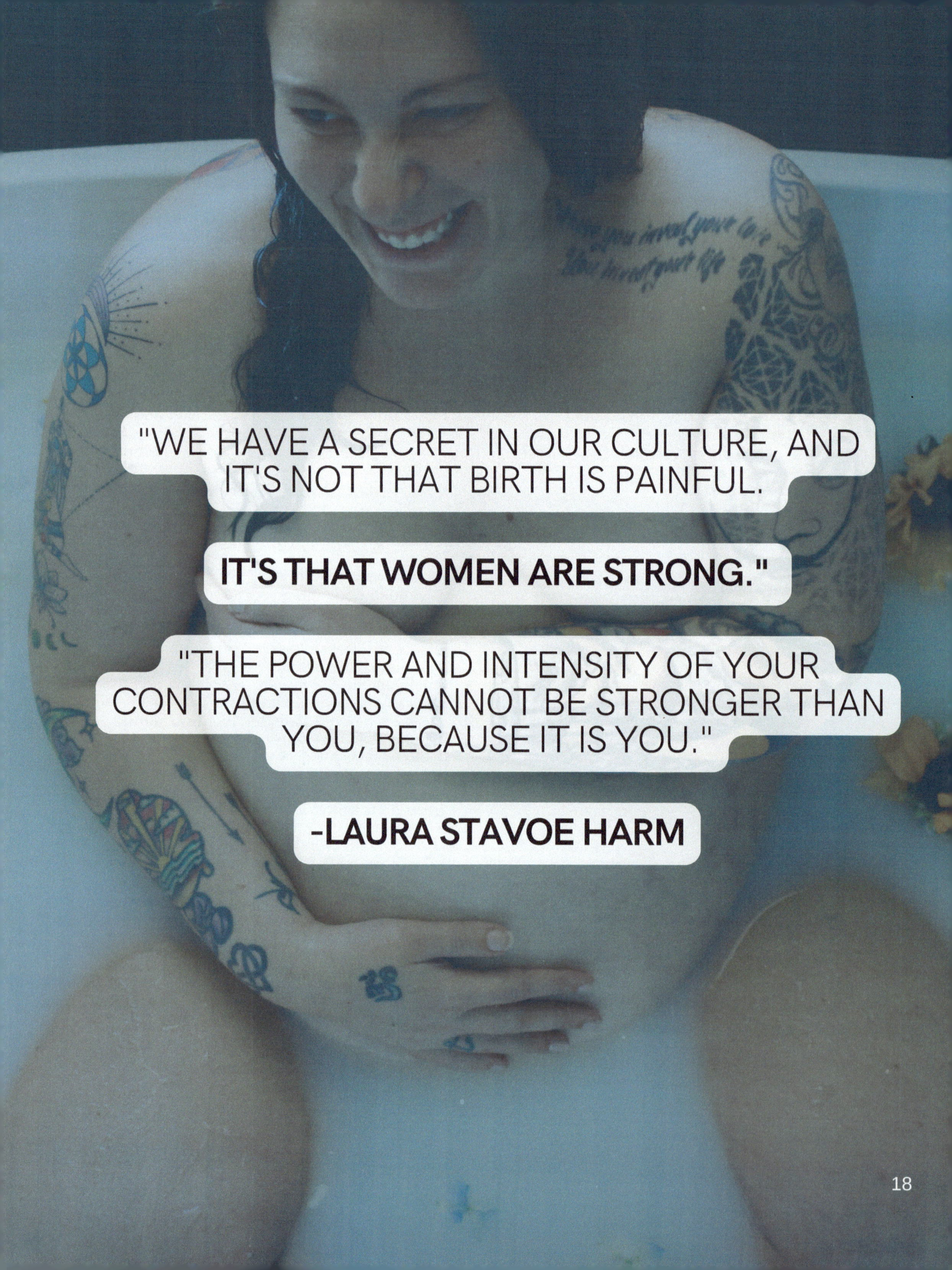

"WE HAVE A SECRET IN OUR CULTURE, AND IT'S NOT THAT BIRTH IS PAINFUL.

IT'S THAT WOMEN ARE STRONG."

"THE POWER AND INTENSITY OF YOUR CONTRACTIONS CANNOT BE STRONGER THAN YOU, BECAUSE IT IS YOU."

-LAURA STAVOE HARM

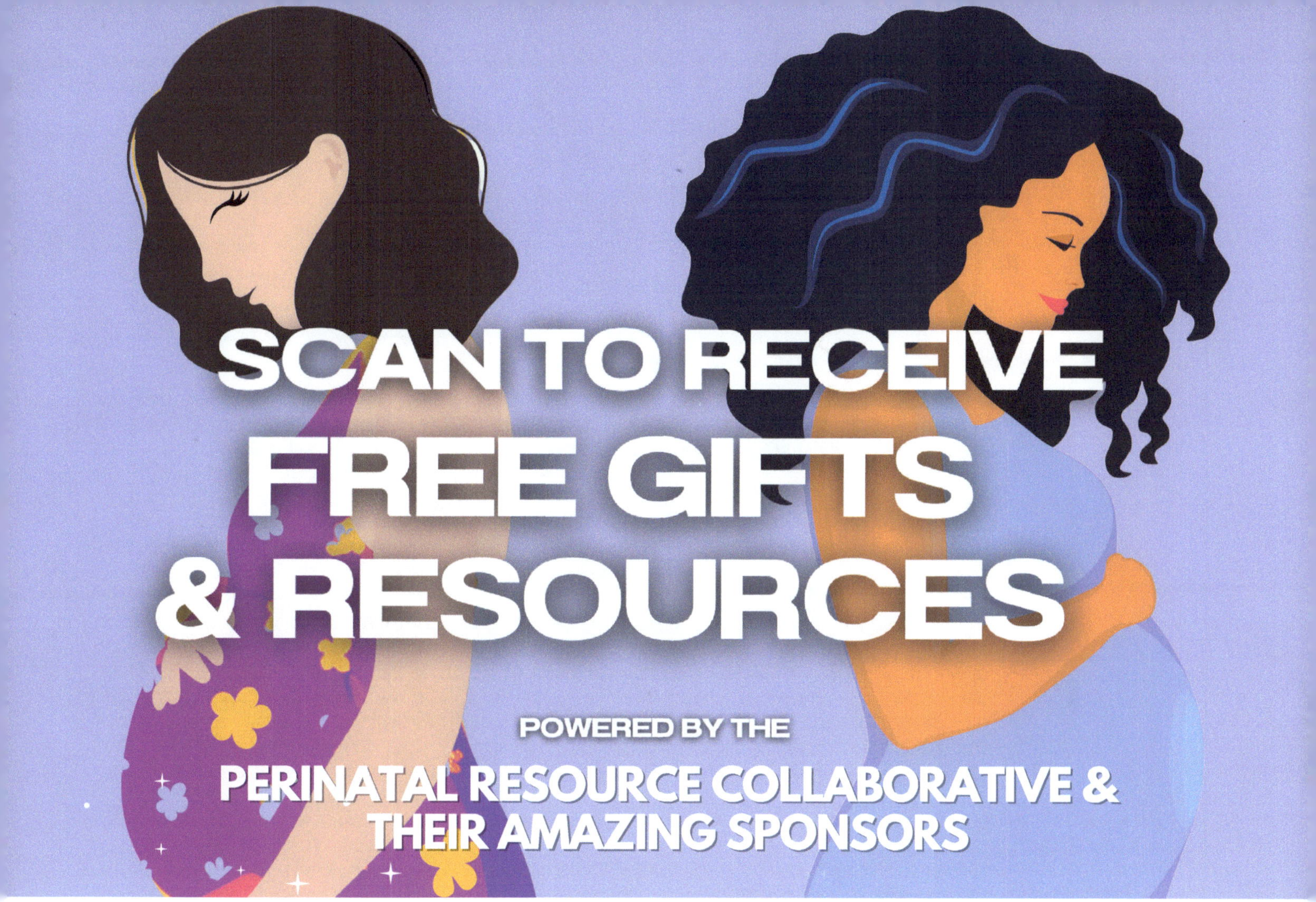

SCAN TO RECEIVE FREE GIFTS & RESOURCES

POWERED BY THE

PERINATAL RESOURCE COLLABORATIVE & THEIR AMAZING SPONSORS

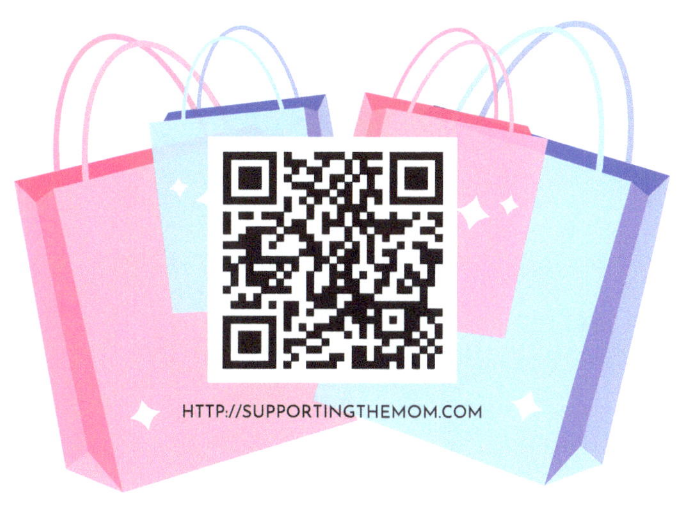

JOIN THE SUPPORTED MOMS CLUB &
FILL OUT THE SURVEY FOR FREE GIFTS AND DISCOUNTS
CONTRIBUTED IN PART BY MEMBERS OF THE
PERINATAL RESOURCE COLLABORATIVE
AND OUR SPONSORS

Optimize Your Body for Home Birth

By Rachael Van Schoick

Most women think about preparing for birth, they focus on creating the perfect birth plan. Choosing what their environment looks like, putting together a support team and really visualizing the birth in explicit detail. Don't get me wrong these things ARE crucial to the birth experience, however, what if I told you that preparing your body is just as critical as planning for the experience? How your body functions, moves, and aligns can directly impact how smooth your baby can navigate through the pelvis with ease and flow. Here are five key factors about your body that can make for a smoother home birth experience.

1. Focus on Pelvic Balance This means creating an environment for the pelvis to be as level as it can be. Creating strength surrounding the pelvis can be a great way to ensure stability in the pelvis and maintain optimal alignment. Simple exercises like, Core Activations, Squats, Sidelying leg lifts, and working the adductors can benefit you greatly here. Along with stretching muscles like the psoas to relieve tension and maintain that balance. Quick Tip: Try implementing these exercises early on to maintain the stability of your pelvis throughout your entire pregnancy.

2. Strengthen and Relax Your Pelvic Floor The ability to contract AND relax your pelvic floor is KEY. During labor, a tight pelvic floor can create resistance, making it harder for your baby to descend. Locating a professional to help you gauge if you have tightness or weakness in your pelvic floor is best, so you can understand which part of a pelvic floor contraction you may need the most or not. Actionable Step: Practice 360 breathing to connect with your pelvic floor. Inhale deeply towards your pelvic floor visualizing your pelvic floor softening and opening. Exhale and feel your pelvic floor gently lifting back into place. The ability to do this contraction without the help of accessory muscles like your glutes, adductors, or extreme contraction of your core is vital here.

3. Master Breathing Techniques Breathing is your greatest ally during pregnancy and labor. Proper breathing helps reduce tension, manage pain, and keep you calm. Even though the baby is growing and taking up more space, it is extremely important to start working on your breath now and creating space. Start practicing techniques like inhaling down towards your pelvic floor and exhaling to lift the abdominals and pelvic floor together. Pro Tip: Combine breathing with visualization. Picture your body opening like a blooming flower with each breath. When it comes to pushing we want to exhale using our abdominals to aid our uterus to help bring the baby down. This is NOT bearing down on the pelvic floor, your pelvic floor should be able to relax as you are doing this.

4. Build Strength and Endurance Labor is often compared to running a marathon, so building endurance is key. Focusing on strengthening our entire body in alignment is crucial. The more interconnected our body is during this time the less our body has to work during labor. Focus on low-impact, functional movements that mimic the positions you'll use during labor. Exercise Idea: If one of the positions you want to attempt to give birth is on all fours, then you should be practicing that position and building strength there to support you so you can maintain the position for an extended period of time. You can also use a birthing ball in this position as well to help hold you up.

5. Prepare for the Unexpected Birth is unpredictable, even with the best preparation. Preparing your body also means preparing your mind to adapt to unexpected challenges. Trust that the work you've put into your physical readiness will support you, no matter how your birth unfolds. Mindset Shift: Incorporate affirmations into your daily routine, like: "My body was made to birth this baby," or "I am flexible and prepared for anything that comes my way." Another example can be to make yourself a powerful playlist that keeps you calm and motivated and repeat those affirmations to yourself.

Conclusion A successful home birth isn't just about the setting; it's about your connection to your body. By focusing on alignment, relaxation, strength, and endurance, you'll enter labor feeling empowered and prepared. Remember, this is your journey, and every step you take to prepare is an act of love for yourself and your baby. Are you planning a home birth and want more guidance on how to prepare your body? Download my free guide on "Optimal Birth Prep" or schedule a consultation to create a personalized plan that supports your birth goals.

My "Power in Postpartum" program is here to help you regain strength, boost your confidence, and return to the activities you love. Over 8 weeks, we'll focus on exercises tailored to your needs, supported by professional guidance and a community of moms just like you. With a blend of core activation, strength work, ELDOA, and mindful movement, you'll heal faster, feel stronger, and be ready for anything.

Join us today and start your journey towards a stronger, healthier, and happier you!

Learn more about the Power in Postpartum program and sign up now!

https://www.alignmovement.com/power-in-post-partum-get-info/

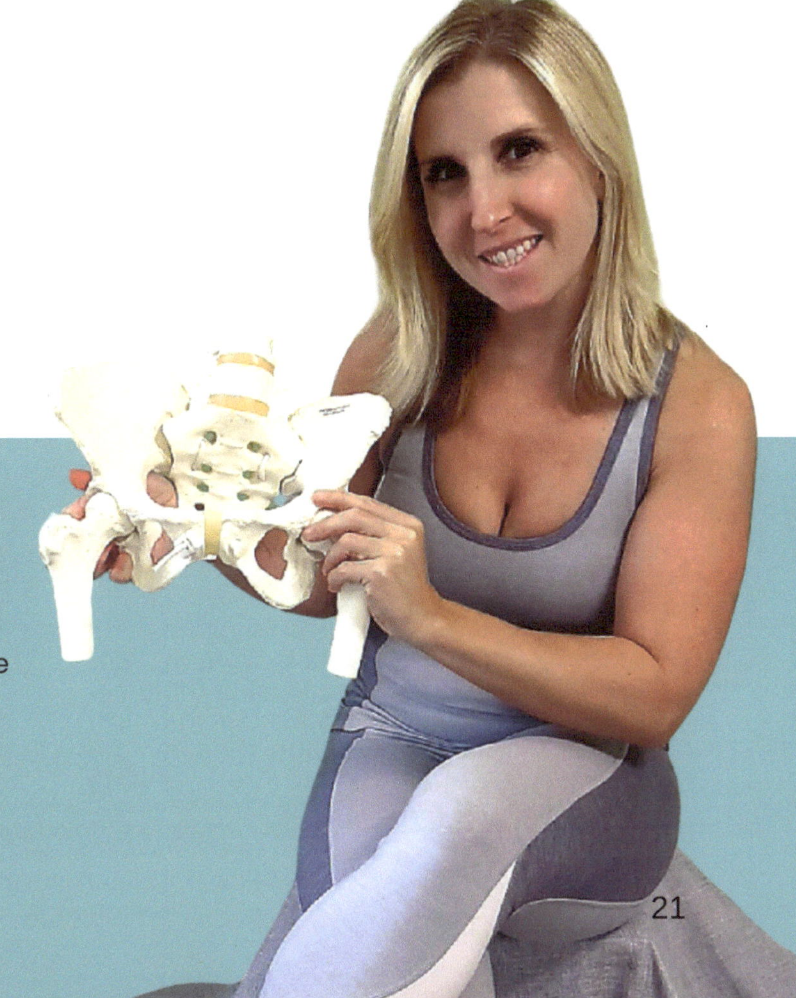

Rachael Van Schoick

Align Movement
LMT, Birth Doula, Prenatal and Postpartum Exercise
Specialist, SomaTrainer and ELDOA Trainer
New Jersey Based but Available Online

@alignmovement_therapy
https://www.alignmovement.com/

Home Birth Sets the Stage for a Healthy Life

By Lesley Franco LM, CPM

Giving birth is one of the milestone events in a woman's life, and the kind of birth a woman has leaves an imprint on her soul. It also leaves an indelible impression on the baby. A positive birth experience, which includes uninterrupted bonding and breastfeeding, provides the best foundation for healthy child development.

The home birth process often begins with enlisting the help of a midwife for prenatal care, Using a midwife to guide you through this exciting time can be a very different experience than being under a doctor's care. Appointments under midwifery care are unhurried and relaxed, making sure there is plenty of time to answer parents' questions. Careful attention is paid to prenatal nutrition, exercise habits and stress-reduction techniques, as well as any labwork necessary to ensure mom stays low-risk. This holistic approach helps keep both mom and baby healthy and minimize risk of complications.

When the time comes to plan for birth, some expectant parents are afraid to leave the perceived "safety" of the hospital environment. However – statistics show that home birth with a qualified attendant is as safe as hospital birth for healthy, low-risk women with adequate prenatal care. Most of the time, there is no need to medicalize the birth process. When a woman honors the rhythm of her body, her unique experience will unfold naturally.

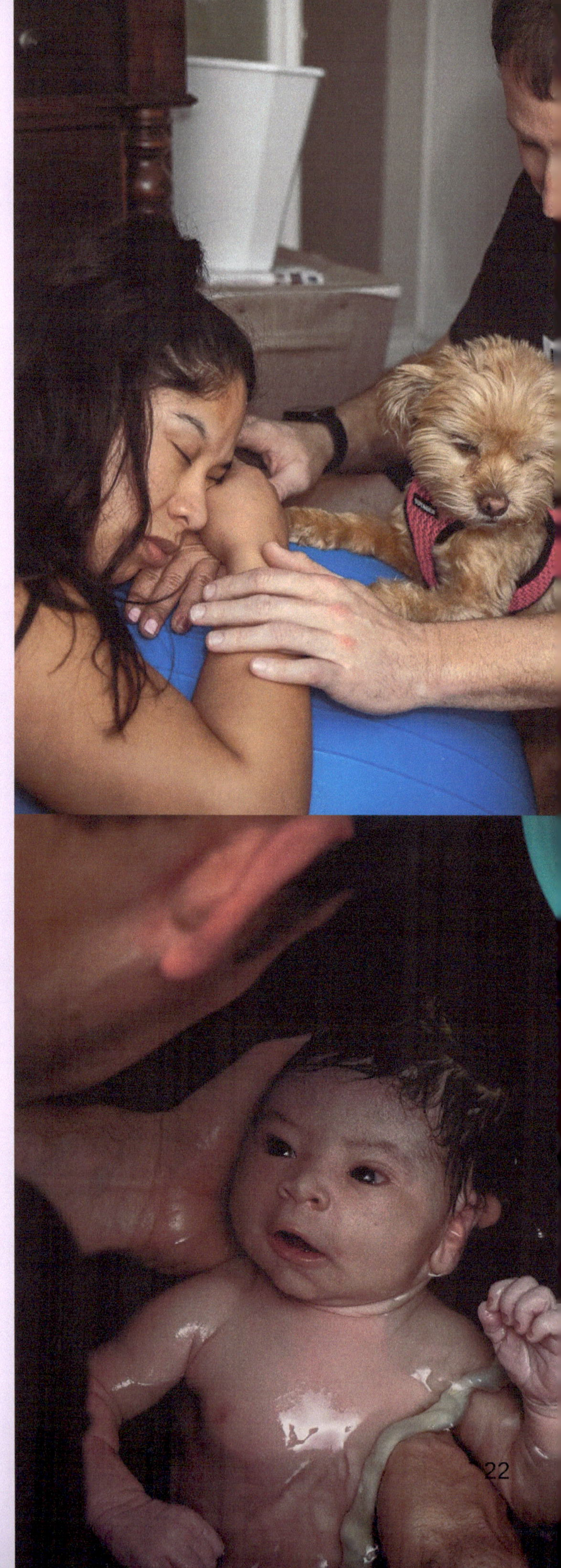

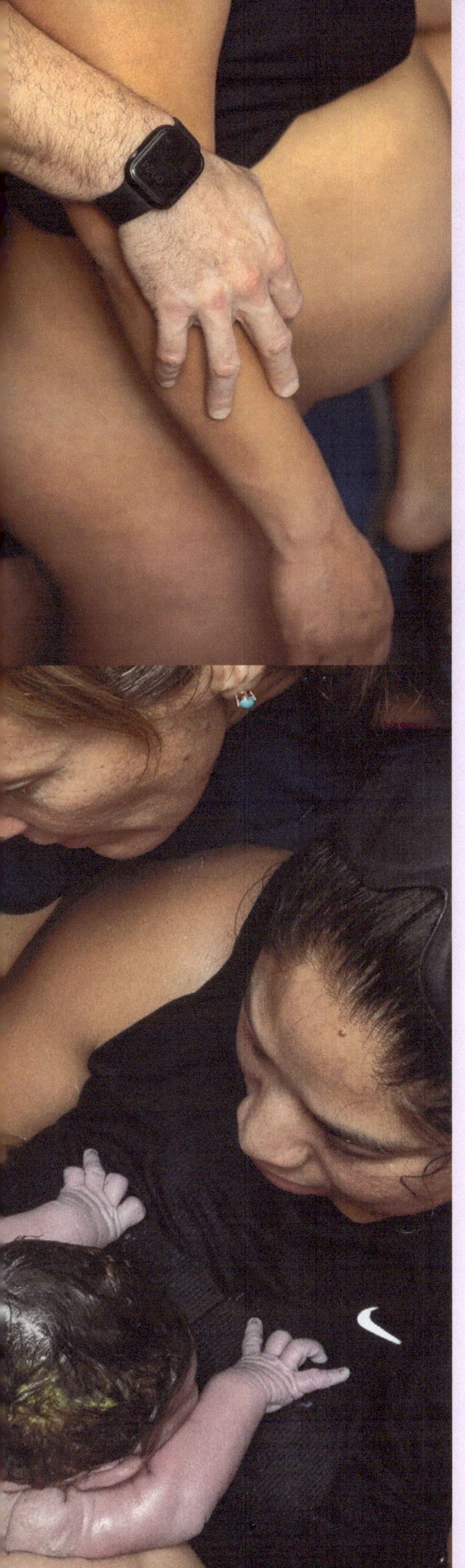

For those of you considering home birth, and others curious about the process, here are some of the advantages of this birthing approach:

- At home, birthing people can labor and deliver in the privacy and comfort of their own familiar environment, with the support of loved ones, and the freedom to utilize any positions or attire they find most comfortable.

- The laboring person maintains control over mostly everything impacting their labor and birth. Meeting their needs is the only focus of all support people present. Nothing is done without consent. The parents and their care provider have established a relationship based on mutual trust and respect.

- Labor is encouraged to progress normally, without interference or unnecessary interventions. Midwives are specialists in physiological labor in the out-of-hospital environment, while obstetricians are surgeons who are trained to look for pathology.

- During labor, the woman is encouraged to eat, drink, walk, change positions, make noise, use the shower or tub for relaxation etc...

- Caregivers are invited guests in the birthing person's home. They can also invite anyone additional they desire for support – such as family members, friends, siblings – even pets. All invited should be mindful, however, that if all that attention should prove distracting, the couple may ask for some privacy at any point in the labor.

- The family unit remains intact because there is (usually) no "leaving for the hospital". Their care providers come to them.

- Careful one-on-one care is given by the midwife, assessing the condition of both mother and baby throughout the birth process and immediate postpartum period. Women are supported and encouraged throughout the hard work of labor, giving them the opportunity to be fully present while experiencing such a powerful, life-changing event.

- Bonding is enhanced by a calm transition period in the first "Golden Hour". Cord clamping is delayed, baby is skin to skin, breast/chestfeeding is facilitated by the baby remaining with the mother/birthing person. No one takes the baby away from the parents, and bonding involves siblings and family members who are present.

Each and every baby comes through as pure love – with unlimited potential and endless possibility. Babies are created in love – not fear, and they deserve the opportunity to be born into love – not fear. Birthing at home, in one's own familiar surroundings, offers such an opportunity to lessen birth trauma and create a gentler transition for the newborn. It also allows an opening for enormous personal growth and transformation for each family member who is present. It is a privilege and an honor for midwives to facilitate a gently, peaceful, warm welcome for newborn babies.

In the words of birth advocate Elizabeth Noble, "I believe that when real change occurs in how babies are brought into this world, and in the consciousness with which they are received, the levels of addiction, violence and crime in society will be reduced. It's a matter of starting at the very beginning".

When considering where, and with whom, you will welcome your new baby, meditate on these words from childbirth author Suzanne Arms "If we hope to create a non-violent world where respect and kindness replace fear and hatred, we must begin with how treat each other at the beginning of life – for that is where our deepest patterns are set – from these roots grow fear and alienation, or love and trust".

If you or someone you love is interested in learning more about midwifery care and home birth, I encourage you to find a certified midwife in your area.

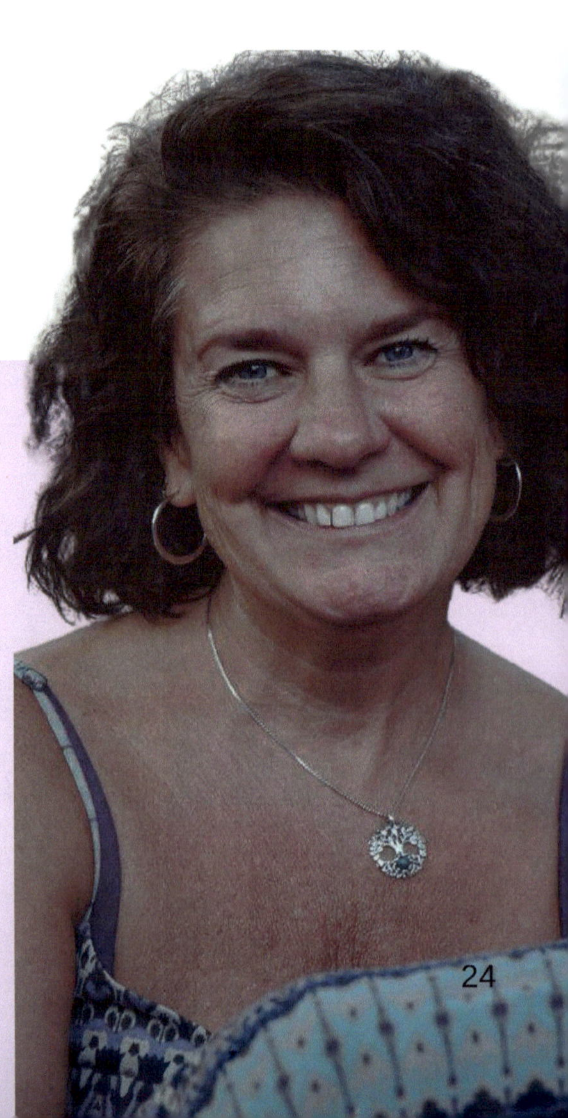

Lesley Franco LM, CPM
is a licensed midwife in Asbury Park, NJ, and proud mama of 3 sons, all born naturally with midwives.

Visit www.soulshinehomebirth.com for more information.

gentlebirth

Meditations App

FOR EXPECTANT MOTHERS

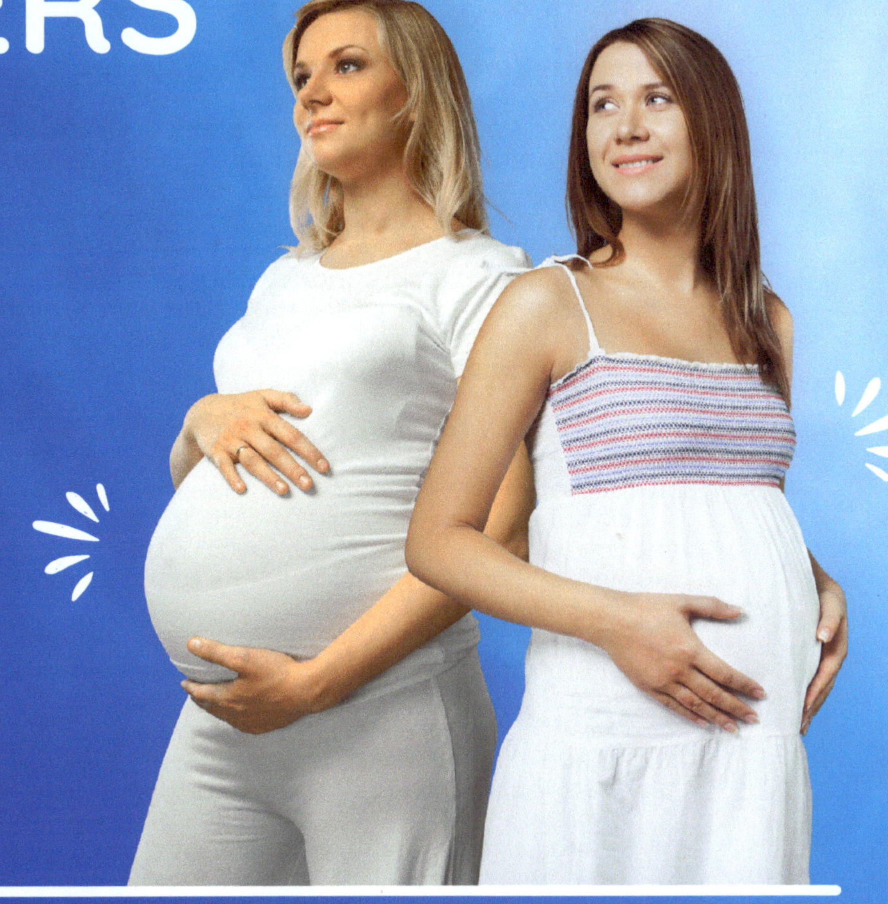

Scan now and unlock premium access at an exclusive price for a limited time!

www.gentlebirth.com

Shattering Two Homebirths Myths So You Are Informed

By Khristee Rich

Homebirths are on the rise in the United States. They have escalated sixty percent from 2016[1]. However, they are hardly the norm representing only two percent of American births. This article will bust some common myths about homebirths and dispel fears so mothers can make informed decisions. For the last five years, I have been researching childbirth around the world through a holistic perspective for my three-book series to empower women. Today, I will dissect two of the most common misunderstandings about homebirths such as 1) homebirths are not safe and 2) you can't have a homebirth if you are thirty-five or older. Plus, I will share perspectives from other countries as well as my research to give greater understanding.

Let's break down these myths step-by-step starting with the most common heard one.

Homebirths are unsafe. They are dangerous.

Contrary to popular belief, homebirths are safe. For hundreds of years, women gave birth at home before the move to hospitals. It was common. It was natural. True, times were different as far as technological advances and medications, but midwifery was a skill that was passed down from women that contained a lot of wisdom. Midwifery care allowed women to move in labor: to sit, stand, or squat. It nurtured them and protected what was natural in pregnancy and birth. Unfortunately, a lot of that wisdom and artistry disappeared once doctors took over. Once birth moved to hospitals, doctors touted themselves as being superior and more prestigious than midwives - do to being medically trained.

Many people who are opposed to homebirths believe that hundreds of years ago, in colonial times, a lot of women were dying in childbirth at home, but there were no statistics. Only slaves were documented because they were considered property. Reports show that their children died mostly from malnutrition in the womb or from not receiving enough nutrition from breastfeeding or sadly, because they were suffocated by their mothers so that they wouldn't have to live in such hardships. Complications at birth were not the number one factor.

Other than that, we do know that in the 1840's in Austria, the rich had their babies at home and only the poor delivered at the hospitals. At that time, the Austrian government developed insurance, and poor mothers were guaranteed to receive financial support if they gave birth at the hospital. However, also at this time, there was a high rate of childbed/ puerperal fever and women were dying after giving birth at hospitals.

Dr. Semmelweis, director of the maternity ward noticed that there was a stark difference between the mortality rates in the wing lead by midwives versus the wing lead by obstetricians. Women were dying four times greater in the wing lead by doctors. He observed both sides and discovered that midwives always washed their hands before working with pregnant women and doctors were often darting from researching cadavers to delivering babies without washing their hands. Although, this was before the discovery of germs in science; midwives intuitively knew to be clean for mothers whereas doctors were spreading germs and causing fatalities.

Today, many obstetricians still view pregnancy and birth more like a pathology than a natural process. They often perform interventions such as episiotomies, forceps, IVs, internal fetal monitors, medications, and try many methods to speed up labor instead of allowing it to happen naturally in its own time. Birth complications and trauma are on the rise. Cortisol and adrenaline are not beneficial at birth and are often activated during hospital births when women feel fearful and pressured to make decisions quickly. Unfortunately, the United States has some of the highest maternal mortality and morbidity rates in the developed world. Most complications and fatalities happen in hospitals, not at home. In addition, the cascade of hospital interventions and medications contributes to higher rates of C-sections. Whereas the Netherlands has one of the highest rates of homebirths in the world, thirty percent of all their births[1] and has some of the best birth outcomes in the world.

You can't have a homebirth if you are thirty-five or older.

Geriatric pregnancies and advanced maternal age are terms that are described as being high-risk for women thirty-five and older in the Unites States. These terms are loathed by women and not only that, this spreads unnecessary fears that it is dangerous to be an older mom and that complications are expected.

According to well-renowned Peruvian OB/GYN, Dr. Antonio Lévano, birth reports state that complications are only slightly higher for older women. About ninety percent of older women will not experience any feared issues. The main consideration should not be age but if a woman is healthy. If women are obese or have chronic conditions prior to pregnancy or develop chronic conditions in pregnancy that are left untreated, these factors can result in birth complications. But if women are healthy, a homebirth is not a risk. It is an option.

Many women who I interviewed were over thirty-five and they had safe, empowered homebirths and were so glad they chose it.

To prepare for a homebirth, I suggest that women prioritize their health before pregnancy to minimize developing health conditions in pregnancy or birth complications, treat health conditions during pregnancy promptly if they arise, and do plenty of research on homebirths so that they feel emotionally and physically prepared. Interview midwives and doulas to get a clear idea if they are the right fit and prepare your home for your comfort with anything from music, candles, a birthing tub, mood lights to essential oils. Also, as a precaution have a Plan B, just in case. Know where the nearest hospital is, how many minutes away, and if they accept transfers. Even if your desires are to birth at home, sometimes it is medically necessary to go to the hospital. Therefore, it is important to have these conversations with midwives and family to make sure they are on board for your and your baby's health. Unfortunately, some midwives are against hospital births and will not do birth transfers. Some are not able to practice at hospitals and therefore, mothers would find themselves without their care once they transfer. Still, it is best to know this ahead of time to prepare.

There is a reason why homebirths have risen over the last five years. Conscious women choose homebirths.They have done their research. They have heard about other women's experiences and have decided what is best for them. Homebirths connect women to their power. They trust their bodies, their support team, and the process. They feel comfortable in their homes. Women have been birthing for centuries, so release your fears, plan ahead, and enjoy your birth.

[1] National Geographic [2] Expatica.

For more information on my book and to be informed about other birth myths, follow me on my Web site at www.thedancingcurtain.com

Khristee Rich, *The Dancing Curtain, LLC*

Find her online @khristeerich or www.thedancingcurtain.com
Based in CT In Person & Virtual Services

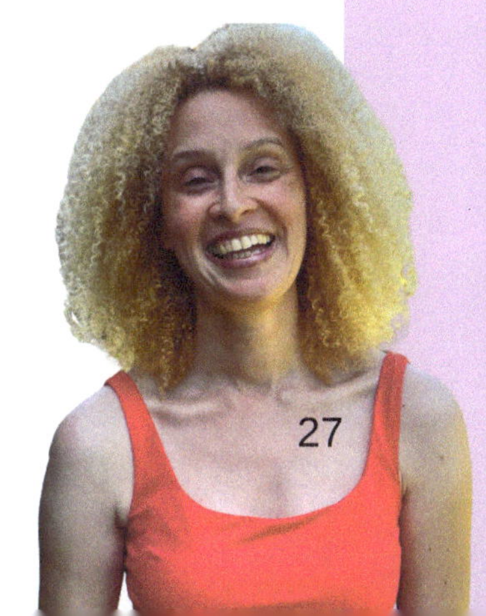

Why Home Birth Could Be the Perfect Choice for Women Over 30

Have you ever felt unheard and dismissed during your journey as a woman when it comes to reproductive health?

Maybe now that you're pregnant you feel this has become more intense. Your health care provider has dismissed everything you said, and because of your "geriatric" age they've made it even more difficult.

It's like you can't catch a break, but now you've been debating on if there might be a different approach to your birth journey that you want.

Homebirth might be the option for you, but every time you think about it, other people's fears stop you. Simply because you're over thirty.

The common thread is that it's too dangerous and something could happen to you or baby, making all the hard work of getting your child to this place for naught...

Well, I'm here to tell you that you might be having the birth you desire, if you open yourself up to that possibility and don't allow others judgements to stop you.

Now, let's drop the age, pretend it isn't a factor (I'll come back to it soon).

There are a lot of reasons why one might choose a home birth - actually I can think of four.

The feeling of control, remember I asked if you were feeling like everything you said was being dismissed, as if someone else was running the show (although you will be giving birth to your child and not them)?

When you're in control you can create a calming environment which can provide you a less stressful birth... possibly giving you more ease then if you were in a hospital. Besides that you'd be able to choose your birthing positions and include any of those personalized touches that you could possibly be denied in the hospital. Such as aromatherapy and music.

Secondly, there is another form of safety and trust when birthing at home. If you choose unassisted or assisted with midwives you'll find that your voice is being heard more often than if you choose another route of giving birth.

By Elisabeth van der Wilt

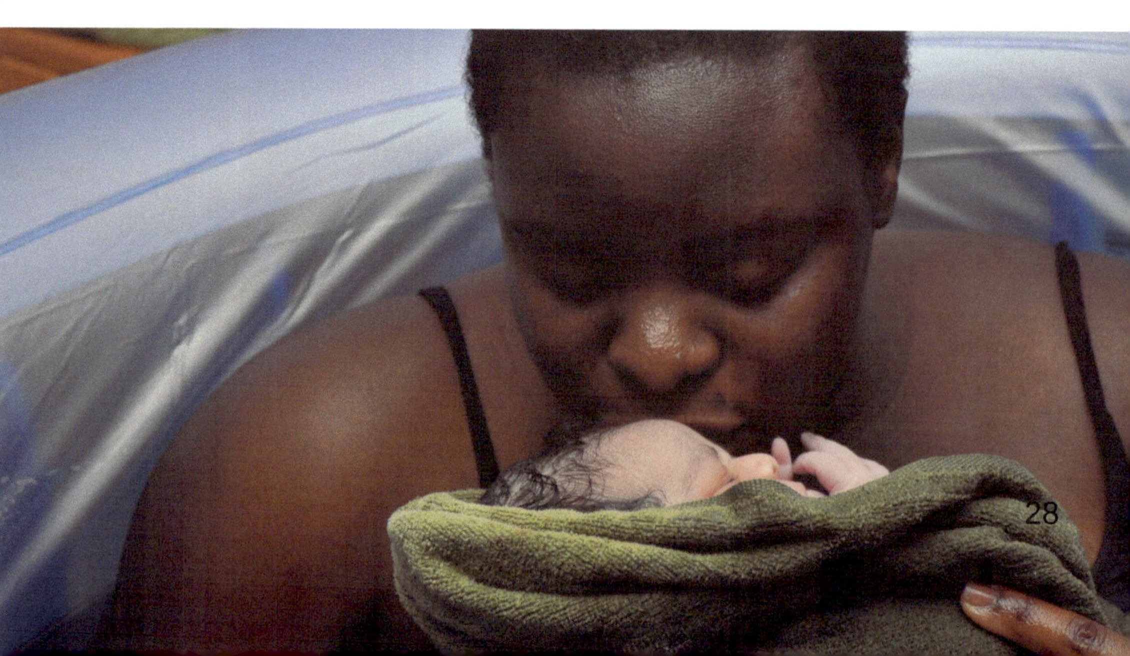

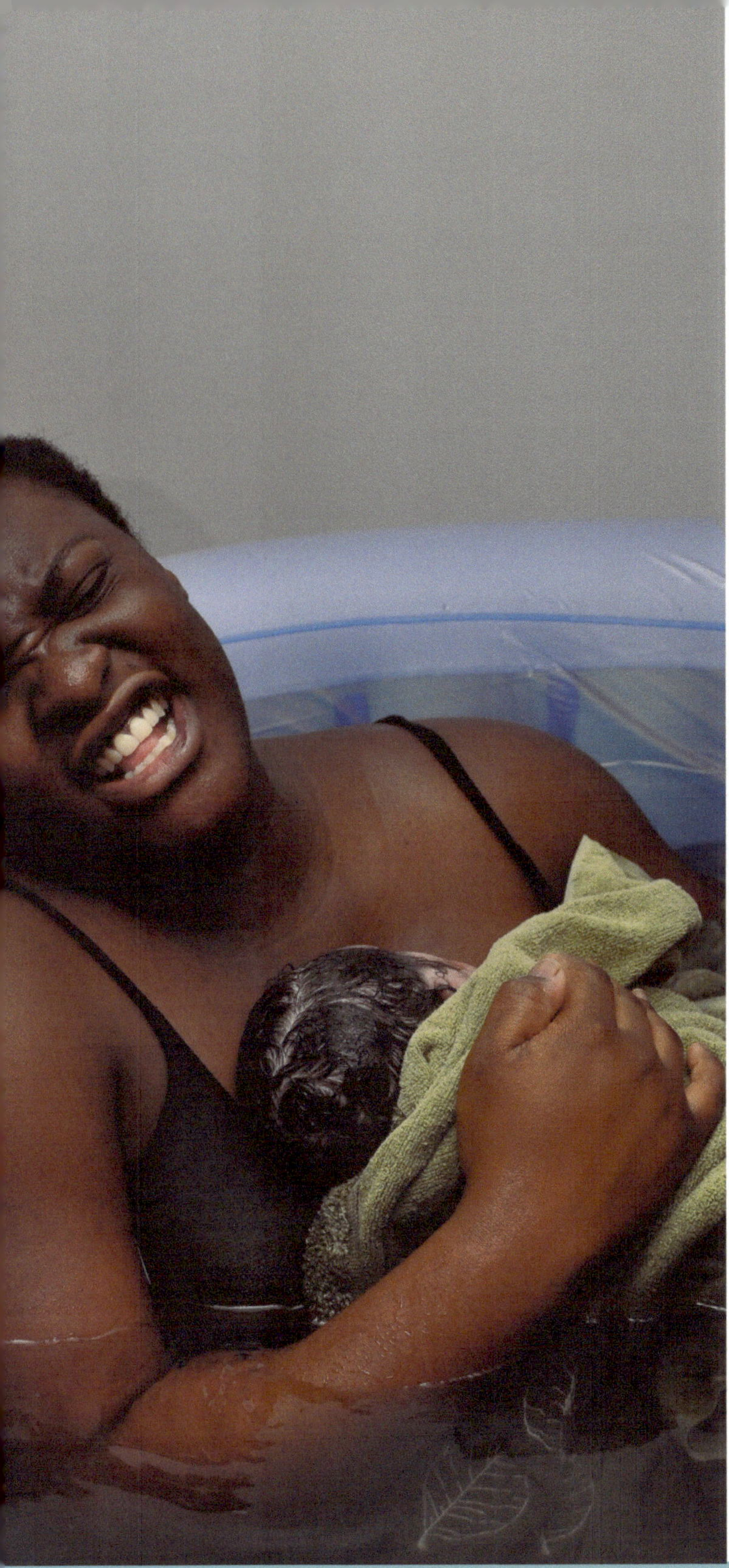

There are also a lot of natural healing values when it comes to home birth. These holistic methods have fewer medical interventions and the ability to follow your body's cue is true. Though, I admit a big con that a lot of women complain about is the lack of pain meds, so before choosing home birth determine what pain coping techniques you'll be learning and attempting.

Lastly, home births are known for being a family-centered care approach. If you currently have other children, or even if you just have a partner, the focus is more on intimately fostering connection and comfort.

If your first thought is I can't have a homebirth because I'm over the age of thirty, then hopefully this article can change your mind. You're more than safe to have a baby at home (age is really just a number, in this case as well).

Having a birth team that you trust and advocate for your safety, and preparing for the what-if's can create the birth environment you want and need to deliver your baby safely in your home.

So a word of the wise would simply be, find out what YOU truly need and want from your birth, ensure you are listening to not only the negative birth stories, but the positive ones as well. Lastly, believe in yourself, if you believe you can do this, then trust me you can and you will.

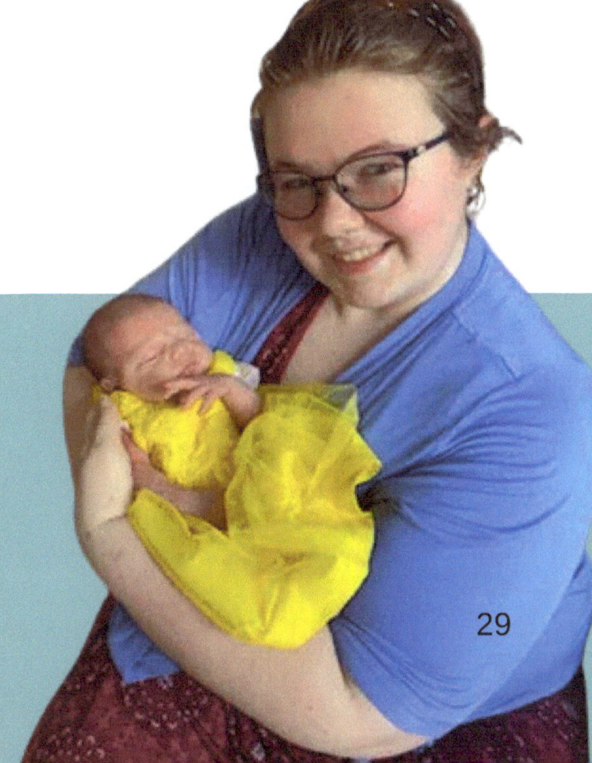

Lisa van der Wilt, *Fruitful Womb Doula Services*
Certified Birth, Postpartum, and Fertility Doula, Birthkeeper,
 Menopause Coach and Advocate, PLC

@fruitfulwombdoula https://fruitfulwomb.ca/
Based in Canada

The Freedom and Empowerment of Sacred Freebirth

By Lalita Love

Free What? You may have heard of the term " freebirth" and asked yourself "what the heck is that?" Well, if you're not up to date on the latest hippy dippy lingo "crunchy" mamas like myself use, no worries. This article is for you!

Freebirth is the term often used to describe the process of giving birth (rather at home or otherwise) without medical assistance. It is a highly personal, deeply spiritual, truly empowering, and unique opportunity for those who choose to experience this form of childbirth! Also, it can be a great alternative option for those who have had traumatic experiences in a traditional hospital setting! The choice to freebirth is often linked to a profound respect for the body's natural and innate ability to give birth without medical interventions. Still, as a woman who has freebirthed twice, I can personally attest that thoughtful consideration and proper preparation, must be taken into account before one embarks on this self-appointed initiation into motherhood.

Read on to discover the power of freebirth and how to accurately prepare for one:

Preparing for a Sacred Freebirth

Prenatal Care:
- Trusting Your Body: While regular check-ups with a healthcare provider can offer valuable insights, it's equally important to trust your body's innate wisdom.
- Spiritual Practices: Incorporate practices like meditation, yoga, or journaling to connect with your inner strength and cultivate a peaceful mindset.
- Education: Educate yourself about the natural birthing process, potential physiological changes, and emergency procedures.
- Exercise: Exercise during pregnancy helps the body optimally prepare for labor, delivery and postpartum.

Creating a Sacred Space:
- Birth Sanctuary: Prepare a serene birthing space that feels nurturing and supportive.
- Natural Elements: Incorporate natural elements like candles, crystals, aromatherapy, or plants to create a calming atmosphere.
- Positive Affirmations: Surround yourself with positive affirmations and visualizations to empower your birthing journey.

Building a Support Network:
- Trusted Companions: Choose supportive loved ones who can provide emotional and physical comfort during labor.
- Online Communities: Connect with other women who have chosen unassisted home birth for shared experiences and advice.

Birth Kit: Gather the essential supplies needed for a home birth. Include supplies for postpartum care such as medicine for afterbirth pains.

Empowering Aspects of Freebirthing:

- Bodily Autonomy: Freebirth allows women to make informed decisions about their bodies and their birthing process.
- Natural Approach: By choosing unassisted birth, women can experience the natural progression of labor and birth. Thus, avoiding medical interventions like epidurals and inductions which interfere with the body's natural rhythm; and may lead to negative outcomes.
- Personalized Experience: A freebirth setting provides an intimate and personalized environment, reducing feelings of stress and anxiety.
- Mind-Body Connection: Freebirth may allow women to connect with their bodies and minds on a deeper level, promoting a more spiritual and transformative experience.
- Emotional Healing: For women who have had previous traumatic birth experiences, freebirth can offer a chance to heal and reclaim their birth stories.

Avoidance of Medical Trauma:

- Unnecessary Interventions: Hospital births often involve traumatic medical interventions, such as forceps deliveries, vacuum extractions, or cesarean sections- many of which are unnecessary. *It's important to note that freebirth is not without risks. While many women have successful unassisted home births, it's crucial to be well-informed, prepared, and to have a backup plan in case of emergencies
- Loss of Control: In a hospital setting, women may feel a loss of control over their bodies and the birthing process, leading to feelings of helplessness and fear.
- Medical Gaslighting/ Coercion: Some women report feeling dismissed or disbelieved by medical professionals, contribute to a negative birthing experience.
- Racism: Many women of color especially black and indigenous women experience racism that leads to inadequate care and/or death.

Myth-Busting with a Spiritual Perspective
- Myth: Unassisted birth is risky and dangerous.
- Fact: It's important to be aware of potential risks. Nonetheless, many women have had safe and empowering unassisted births. Trusting your body's innate wisdom and preparing adequately can significantly reduce risks.
- Myth: Unassisted birth is selfish and irresponsible.
- Fact: Many women choose unassisted birth as a deeply personal and spiritual decision, believing it honors the sacred nature of childbirth.
- Myth: Unassisted birth is painful and traumatic.
- Fact: While labor can be intense, many women find that unassisted birth allows them to connect with their bodies and the natural rhythm of their labor, leading to a more positive and empowering experience.

Lalita Love

Sacred Waters Holistic Care
Contact her:
cook.llomi@gmail.com

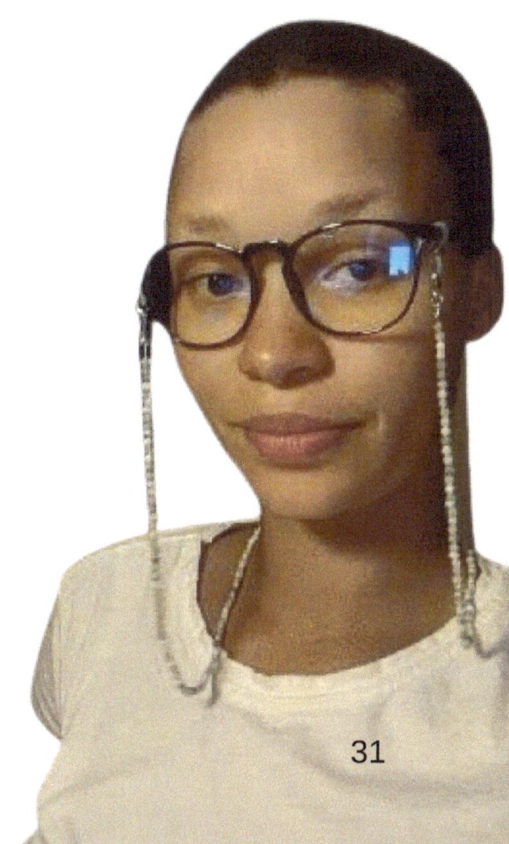

Free birth,
A journey wild and unconfined,
A whirlwind of the spirit,
Combining body, and soul,
Unbound by rules,
A primal rite,
It's the ancient mothers who guide the night,
A creatrix's decree,
Muted prayers and silent pleas,
Cosmic energy,
Ever flowing,
Akashic knowledge ,
It's she who holds the knowing,
No sterile rooms,
No protocols creating gloom,
But a space for grace and love to bloom,
Each breath a mantric wave
Embracing the unknown is a sacred defense,
Through every surge one meets their power,
It could last days,
It could lasts hours,
As life unfolds there is no rush,
Just a rhythmic dance one learns to trust,
An Instinctual force,
A divine feminine design,
A gentle touch,
A loving eye,
A child is born,
The joys of life
A wild and untamed journey,
Welcome to the other side.

-Lalita Love: Sacred Waters Holistic Care

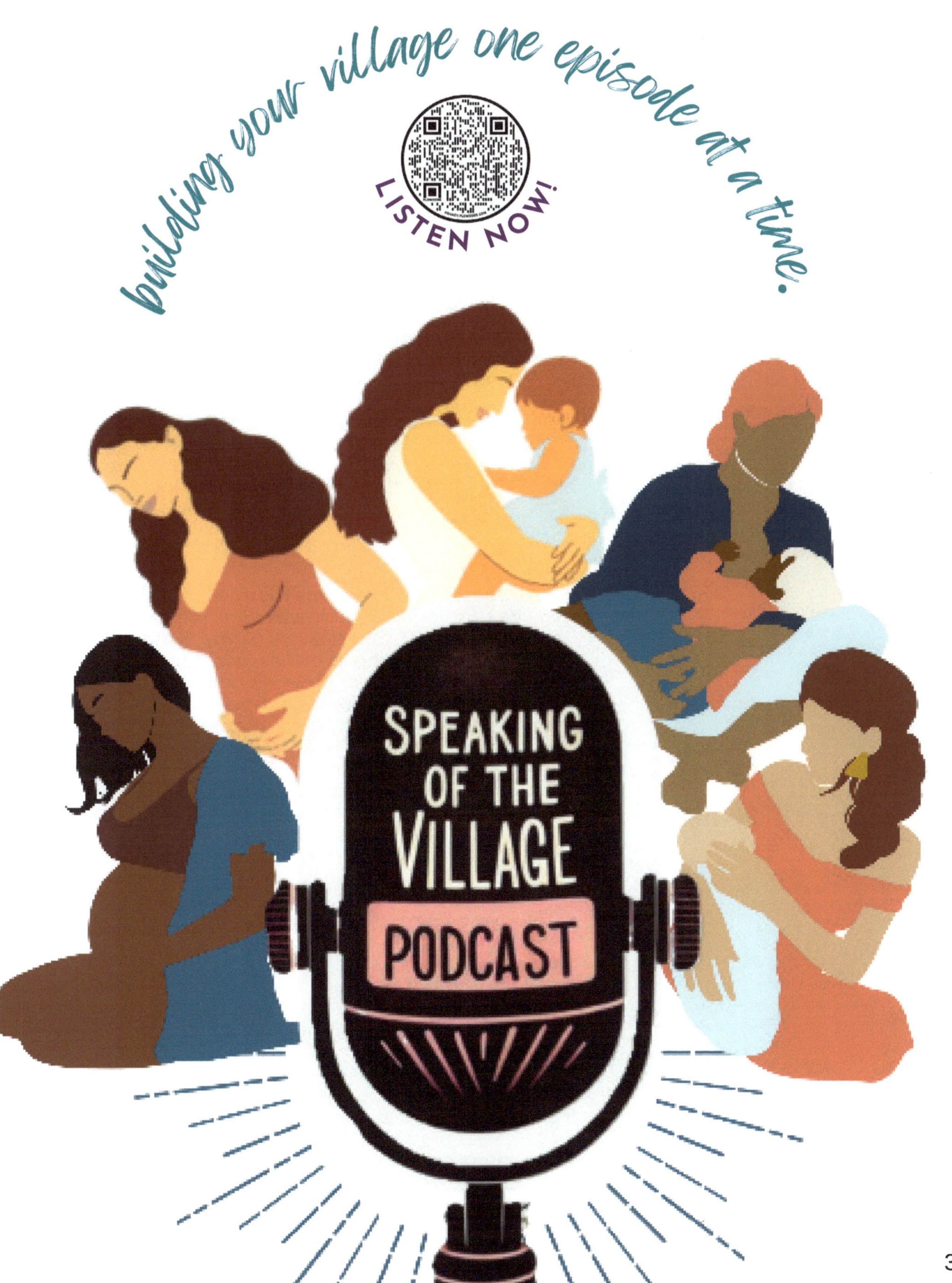

building your village one episode at a time.
LISTEN NOW!
SPEAKING OF THE VILLAGE PODCAST

Is Home Birth For You? Here's What New Moms Need to Know

By Lital Bernstein

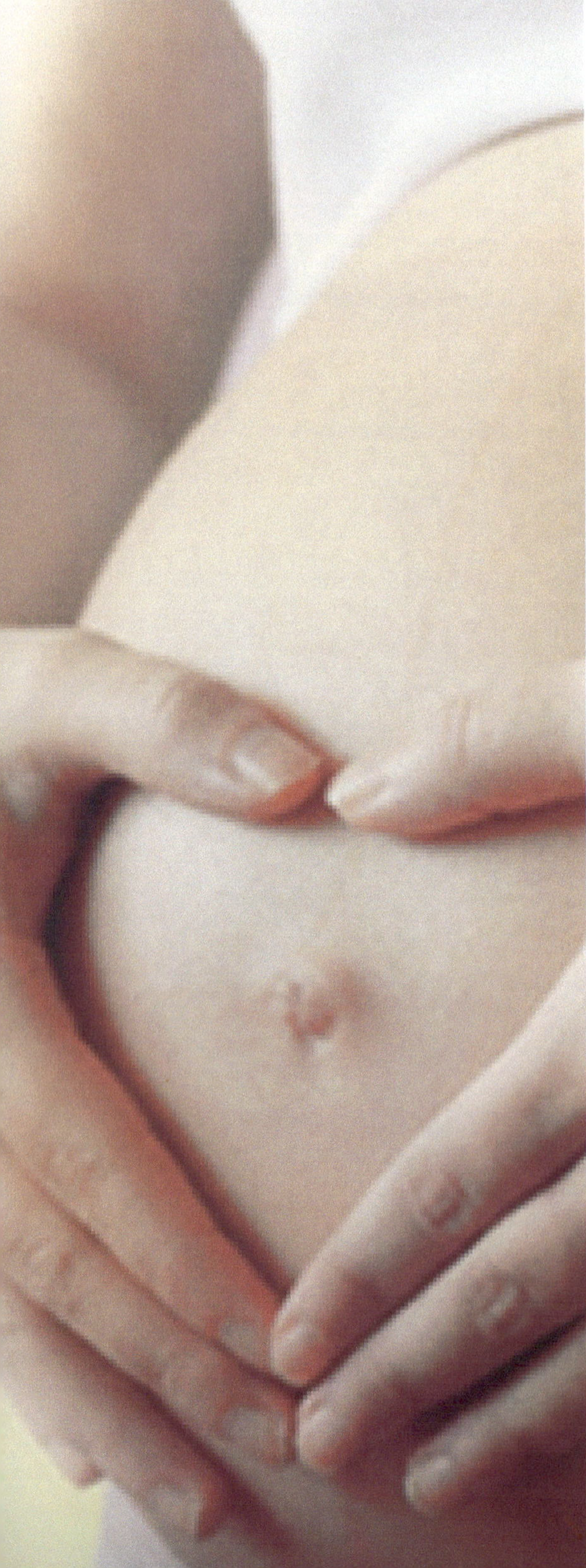

So, you're thinking about having a home birth? That's awesome! With more and more moms-to-be considering the comfort of their own home for this incredible experience, it's no wonder you're curious. Home birth can be a beautiful and empowering choice, but it's also one that comes with a lot of questions and things to think about. Let's dive into what a home birth is all about, the benefits, the challenges, and everything you need to know to make the best decision for you and your baby.

What is a Home Birth?
A home birth is exactly what it sounds like—giving birth in the comfort of your own home rather than a hospital or birthing center. It's a more intimate setting where you can relax and have more control over your birthing environment.

Who's Involved?
When you choose a home birth, you'll typically have a midwife or a team of midwives who are trained to support you through labor and delivery. Some families also choose to have a doula, who provides additional emotional and physical support. These professionals come prepared with everything they need for a safe and smooth delivery, from monitoring tools to emergency supplies.

Why Choose Home Birth?
There are a bunch of reasons why moms might opt for a home birth. Some love the idea of being in a familiar and cozy environment, where they can make their own rules and feel more relaxed. Others appreciate the flexibility and personal attention they get from their midwives. It's also a great way to involve family in a more meaningful way and create a memorable, personal experience.

The Process:
So, what actually happens during a home birth? Typically, you'll start labor at home, and your midwife will arrive when things get going. They'll help you through the stages of labor, provide medical care as needed, and support you in delivering your baby. After the birth, you get to stay home and settle in with your new little one, with follow-up visits from your midwife to ensure everything is going smoothly.

Choosing a home birth is a big decision and one that's all about what feels right for you and your family. If you're intrigued by the idea of giving birth in a place where you feel most comfortable, a home birth might be worth considering.

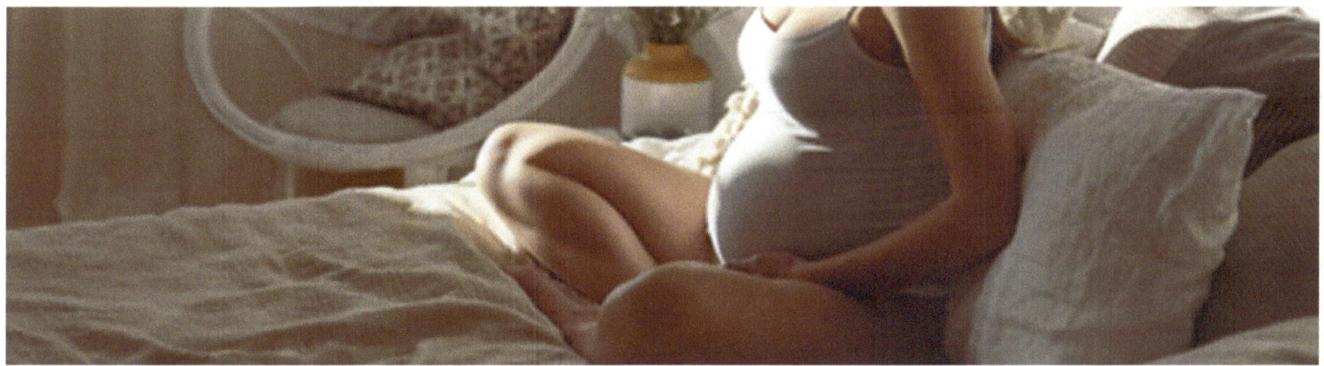

What are the Benefits of a Home Birth?

Home birth is definitely not the path for everyone, but there are some pretty fantastic benefits that make it a great choice for many moms. Here's why you might love the idea of welcoming your little one right at home:

Comfort and Familiarity: One of the biggest perks of a home birth is the comfort of being in your own space. You can create a cozy environment that feels just right for you.You're in your own space, surrounded by familiar things, and you can let your nervous system relax. It's a huge plus to be able to wear your favorite pajamas, have your favorite snacks close by, and be surrounded by things that make you feel cozy and at ease.

More Control Over Your Birth Plan: At home, you have more flexibility with your birth plan. If you want to move around, change positions, or try different comfort measures, you can do so without the constraints of a hospital setting. You're in charge of how you labor and deliver, with your midwife supporting your choices. It's a more personalized experience, where you can make decisions about how you want your labor and delivery to go, without the typical hospital routines.

Close Family Involvement: One of the great things about home birth is how it can involve the whole family. Siblings, partners, and loved ones can be present in a more intimate way, which can make the experience even more special. It's a chance for everyone to be part of welcoming the new baby.

Quicker Recovery: After your baby arrives, you get to stay in your comfy home and settle in at your own pace. There's no need to worry about hospital policies or schedules—just you, your baby, and your cozy space. Plus, having your own bathroom and bed can make a recovery a lot easier and more comfortable.

Lower Risk of Unnecessary Interventions: Many moms find that home births come with fewer medical interventions. Because you're in a more relaxed environment, there's often less pressure and fewer routine procedures. Your midwife will focus on supporting you naturally and only recommend medical interventions if absolutely necessary.

Bonding Time: Home birth gives you the chance to bond with your baby right away, without the hustle and bustle of a hospital setting. You can enjoy those first moments together, start breastfeeding, and begin to establish a routine in a relaxed atmosphere

What are the considerations and challenges to consider?

We've talked about the awesome benefits of a home birth, but it's also important to be aware of some potential challenges and considerations. This isn't to scare you away but to make sure you're fully prepared for what's ahead. Here's what you need to think about:

Safety First: One of the biggest things to think about is safety. Home births can be very safe when managed by experienced professionals, but it's crucial to have a well-trained midwife who knows how to handle any situation that might come up. Make sure you're comfortable with their experience and qualifications.

Always Have a Backup Plan: It's always a good idea to have a backup plan just in case things don't go as expected. Your midwife should have a plan for transferring you to a hospital if necessary. Make sure you're aware of the nearest hospital and have a route planned out. It's about being prepared, just in case.

Fears and Misconceptions: There are some common myths about home births, like the idea that they're riskier or that you're all alone. In reality, many moms have safe and beautiful home births with the right support. It's helpful to talk through any fears or concerns with your midwife or a trusted healthcare professional to get the facts.

Space and Supplies: You'll need to prepare your home for the birth. This means setting up a clean and comfortable space for labor and delivery. You'll also need to gather some supplies, like towels, a birth pool if you're planning on water birth, and basic medical equipment. Your midwife will guide you on what's needed, but it's good to be prepared.

Emotional Preparation: Home birth can be an emotional journey, and it's important to be mentally prepared. Talk with your partner, family, or support system about your plans and make sure everyone's on board. You can also do a <u>Healing Circle Meditation</u> to prepare you for that day. It can be a bit of a rollercoaster, so having a solid support network in place can make a big difference.

Recovery Considerations: While recovering at home is comfortable, it also means you'll need to manage your own care and any complications that might arise. Make sure you have support in place for the postpartum period, including help with household tasks and baby care. To have a home birth, you must be 100% sure that it's what you want, understand all the risks, and take responsibility for the decision. It is not for everyone. You must educate yourself thoroughly and trust that this is the right choice for you. This is a very personal decision. If you have any doubts about it, it's better not to choose this route, as those doubts could subconsciously increase your risk.

How to Prepare for a Home Birth?

Find the Right Midwife: Your midwife will be your go-to person for a home birth, so it's crucial to find someone who's experienced and makes you feel comfortable. Do some research, read reviews, and have a few chats to make sure you're on the same page. They'll guide you through the whole process and help you prepare for the birth.

Gather Birthing Supplies & Comfort Items: You'll need to get a few things ready for the big day. Your midwife will give you a list, but common items include towels, a waterproof sheet, and a birth pool if you're planning on a water birth. Stock up on things that make you feel cozy—think pillows, blankets, snacks, and <u>postpartum essentials.</u>

Medical Supplies: Your midwife will bring most of the medical supplies, but make sure you have things like a thermometer, a clean area for the birth, and any specific items your midwife might recommend.

Create a Birth Plan: A birth plan is like your roadmap for the day. It outlines what you'd like to happen during labor and delivery, including your preferences for pain management, who you want present, and any special requests. Share this plan with your midwife so they know exactly how to support you.

Prepare Your Home: Set up a dedicated space for labor and delivery. This could be your bedroom or another cozy spot in your home. Make sure it's clean, comfortable, and ready for you to spend time in. You might also want to set up a "rest and recovery" area for after the birth.

Communicate with Your Support System: Let your family and friends know about your plans. If you want them involved, make sure they understand their role and how they can best support you. It's also a good idea to have a backup plan for childcare or other responsibilities if you need extra help.

Plan for Postpartum Care: Recovery is an important part of the process. Ask for help with household chores, meal prep, and baby care, and stock your postpartum kit for the days and weeks following the birth. Having support in place will let you focus on bonding with your baby and taking care of yourself.

Choosing a home birth can be a beautiful and personal experience, offering you the chance to bring your little one into the world in a setting that's all about you and your family. It's a journey that requires careful planning and support, but it can be incredibly rewarding.

Remember, finding what feels right for you and your baby is the most important thing. If you're drawn to the idea of a home birth, take the time to research, prepare, and connect with the right professionals to make your experience as smooth and positive as possible.

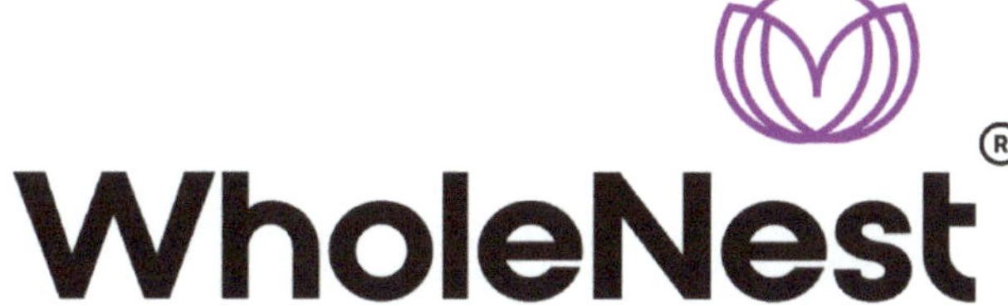

WholeNest started as a solution provider to help every pregnant, and postpartum mom enjoy natural relief and be the best version of themselves to shower the utmost care on their little one. Truly, cannot give what you don't have.

We curated a list of organic essentials with Earth's best natural ingredients, that are hypoallergenic, pregnancy, postpartum, and breastfeeding-safe. Our postpartum care products were initially designed for self-use, but Lital, the Founder, couldn't hold back but offer these wellness essentials to other moms.

Our products, classes, and posts are designed with clear intention, and we combine knowledge, practicality, wisdom, and spirituality to give you the best.

With a multitude of first-hand experiences in various body pains, we thought: Why not create all-around products for everybody that can solve more than just one pain point?
Our nurture from within approach is the backbone of everything we do. Made with you and your family in mind, WholeNest was created to offer multi-functional products that take on the job of several different treatments.

WholeNest is for you. WholeNest is for your family. WholeNest is for everyone.

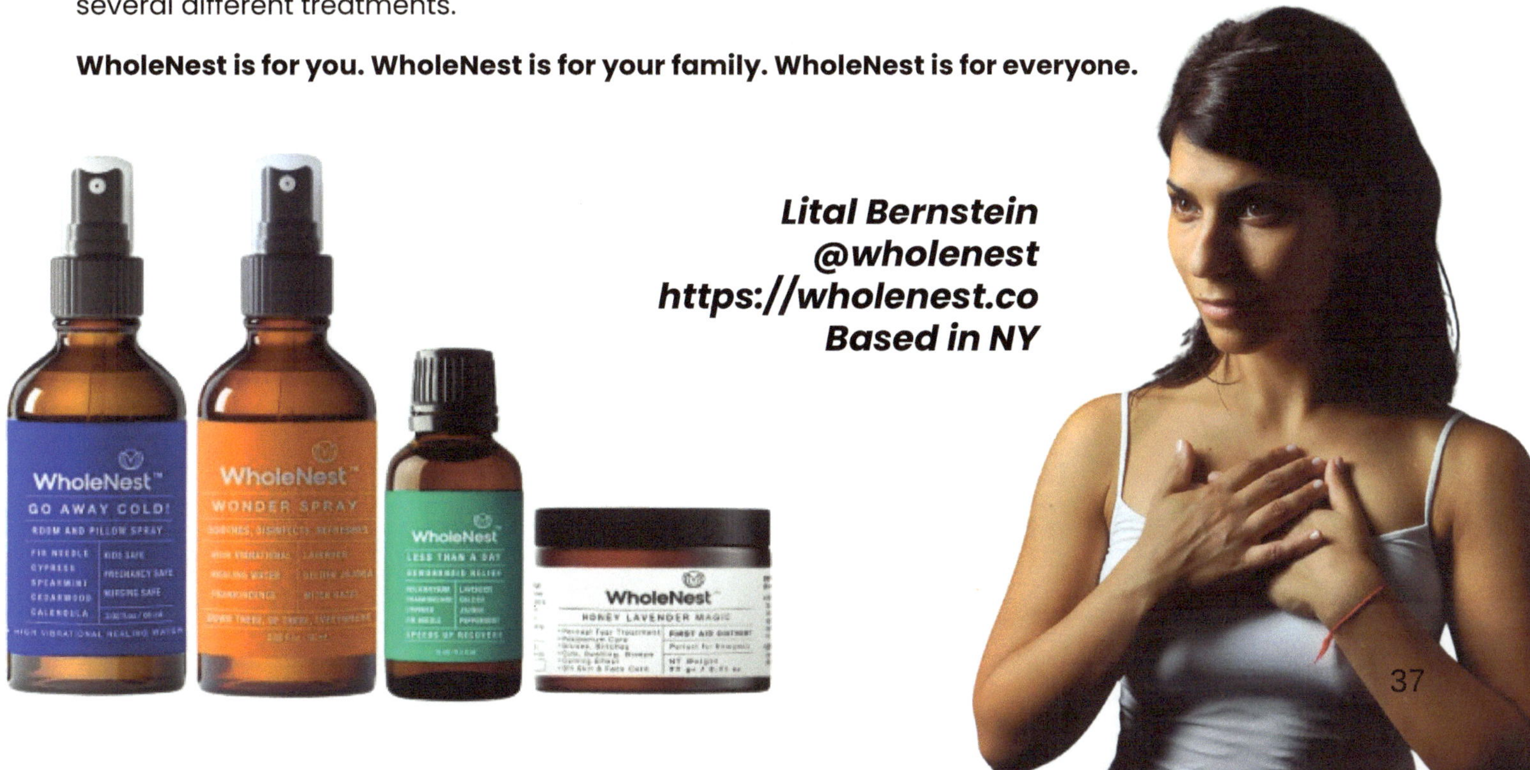

MIDWIFERY CARE
Before & After Birth

By Nicole Harlot

Planning for a homebirth comes with unexpected benefits that are often not associated with the decision. Midwifery care offers numerous benefits during both the prenatal and postpartum periods. Now, these may vary based on location and provider but in my experience, and what I know to be true of CPMs in my area is that their care model is very difference than that of an OB/GYN. Here's a breakdown of some key advantages:

- **Personalized Care:**
  - Midwives provide individualized attention, tailoring care to the specific needs and preferences of the mother.
  - Home visits that are less invasive and more relationship building.

- **Holistic Approach:**
  - Focus on physical, emotional, and social well-being, ensuring comprehensive care.
  - Gives you education and options based on your preferences.

- **Continuity of Care:**
  - Consistent support from the same caregiver throughout pregnancy, fostering trust and understanding. They are on a similar schedule to OB Visits prenatally, but see you many more times in early postpartum than an OB does.

- **Education and Empowerment:**
  - Midwives educate mothers about pregnancy, childbirth, and newborn care, empowering them to make informed decisions.

- **Reduced Interventions:**
  - Emphasis on natural birth processes, often resulting in fewer medical interventions and a more positive birth experience.
  - Understand that cervical checks are not very telling and opt to only do them if absolutely necessary.

- **Support for Natural Birth:**
  - Encouragement and support for natural birthing methods, including home births and water births.

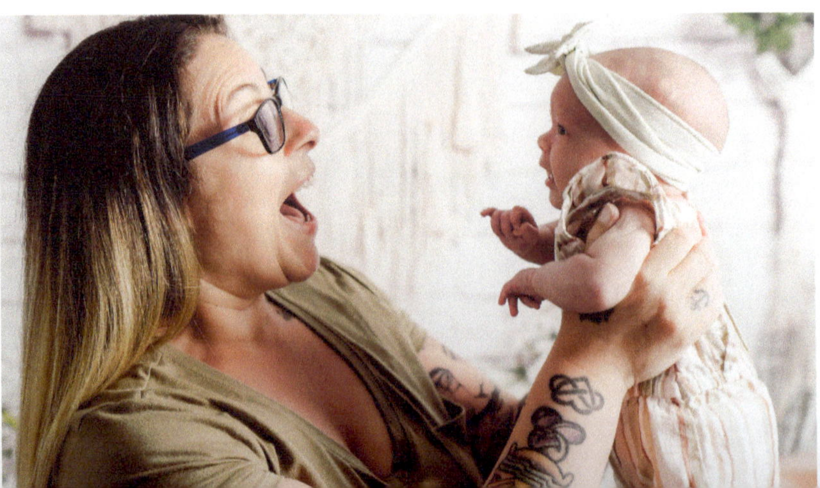

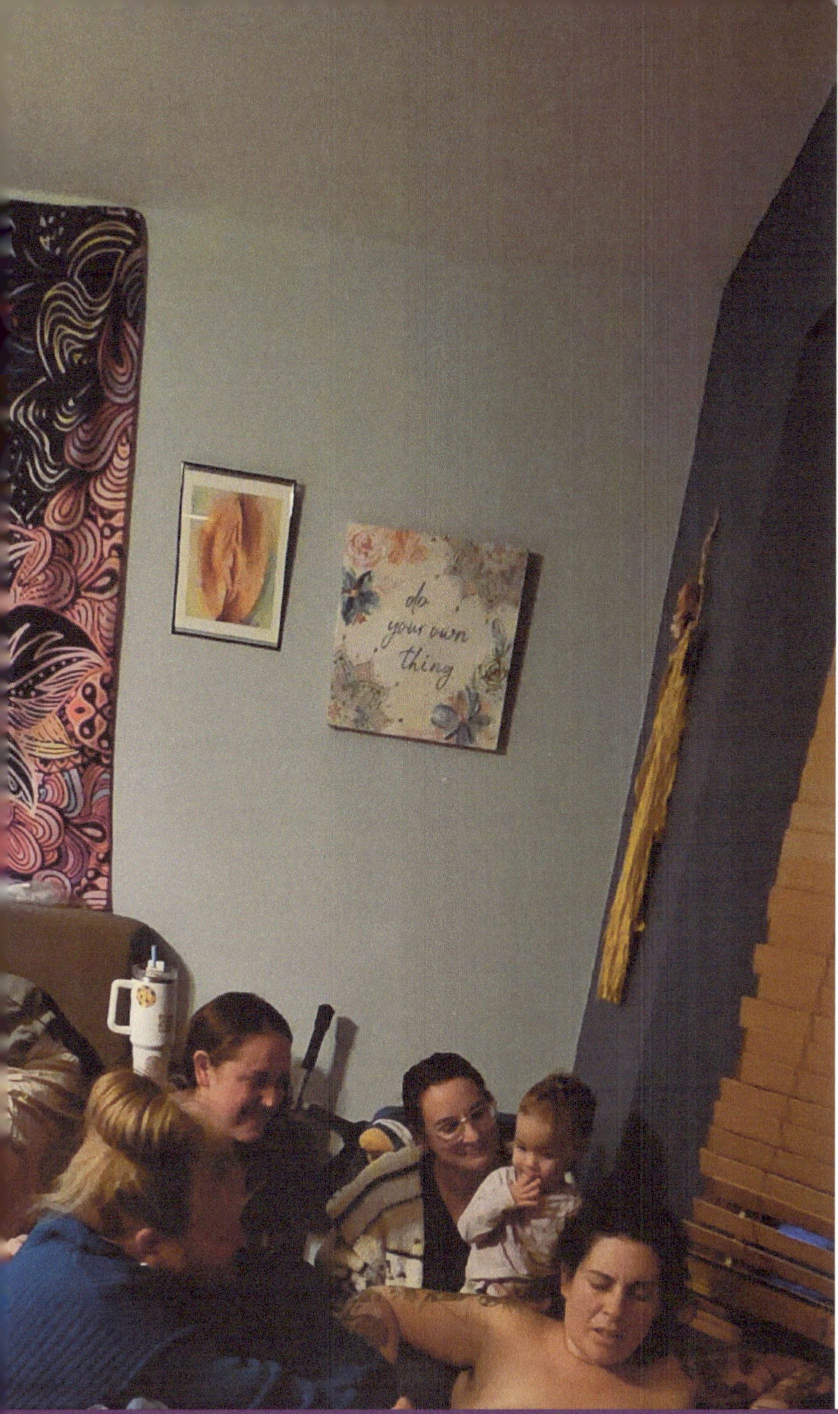

Postpartum Benefits:

- **Postnatal Support:**
    - Continued care and support after birth, helping with recovery and adjustment to motherhood.
    - Check in multiple times, help with newborn care in the early days.

- **Breastfeeding Assistance:**
    - Guidance and support for breastfeeding, addressing challenges and promoting successful nursing.

- **Emotional Support:**
    - Attention to the emotional and mental health of the mother, providing resources and referrals if needed.

- **Family Involvement:**
    - Encouragement of sibling and family participation in care, strengthening family bonds and support systems.

- **Monitoring and Follow-up:**
    - Regular check-ups to monitor the health of both mother and baby, ensuring any issues are addressed promptly.

- **Community Resources:**
    - Connection to other community resources and support groups, fostering a supportive network for new mothers.

Midwifery care is known for its compassionate, patient-centered approach, which can lead to better outcomes for both mothers and babies. How do you feel about the role of midwives in supporting families during these critical periods?

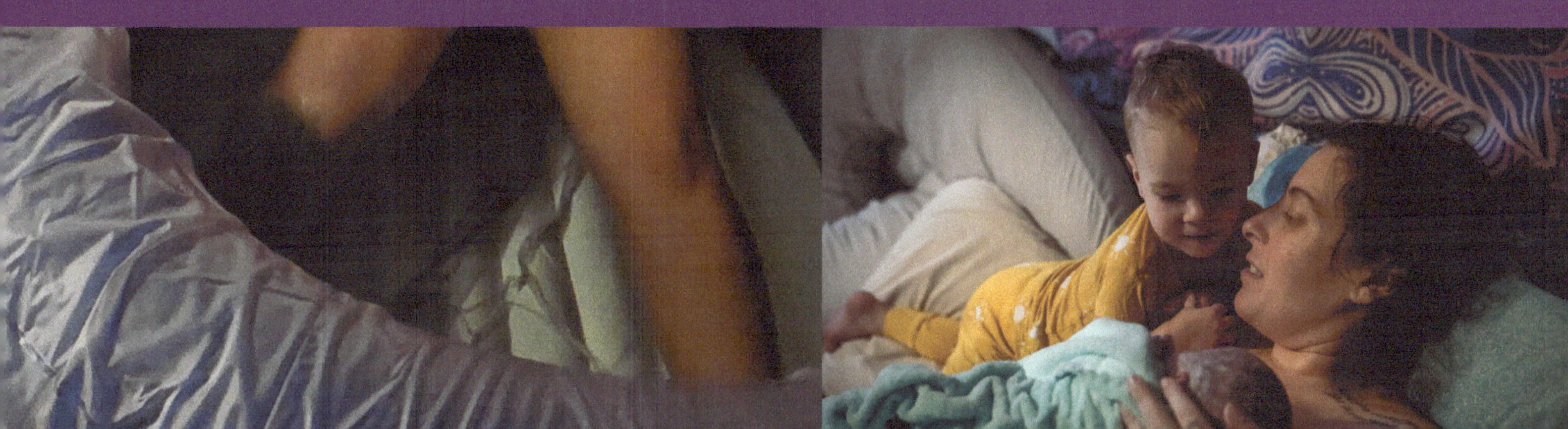

Traditional Postpartum Recovery: Honoring the Sacred Journey.

By Stephenie Ignacio

The postpartum period is a sacred and transformative time, a period that holds great importance in a woman's recovery and well-being after childbirth. Ancient traditions of postpartum care have withstood the test of time —they honor the physical, emotional, and spiritual shifts that accompany the transition to motherhood. Rooted in cultures around the world, these traditions offer more than just rest; they serve as rituals for deep healing, bonding, and nurturing the new mother.

A Holistic Approach to Healing: Traditional postpartum recovery often embraces a holistic view of healing—one that balances the body, mind, and spirit. Unlike the "Bounce Back" ideology that is common in modern postpartum care, traditional practices consider the deeper, often more personal, needs of the new mother. These traditions include physical healing practices, nutritional nourishment, emotional support systems, and community involvement, all guiding the mother through this intense life transition.

From cultures across the globe, we can see various ways of supporting a new mother through her recovery. In many cultures, the postpartum period, often considered a time when the new mother is encouraged to rest and recuperate. She is typically cared for by her family, avoiding the physical and emotional stress that comes with caring for a newborn on her own. This period is meant to restore her vitality, allowing her body to heal fully from childbirth while also building strength for the demanding months ahead.

Nourishing the Body: One of the core elements of traditional postpartum care is nourishing the mother's body. After the intense physical effort of childbirth, a woman's body needs proper nourishment to regain strength. Traditional postpartum practices often involve consuming warm, nutrient-dense foods designed to replenish the body's energy reserves, promote milk production, and restore the blood supply.

Foods like soups, broths, and herbal tonics are vital. These dishes are rich in vitamins, minerals, and proteins that are believed to promote healing, reduce inflammation, and support lactation. In Chinese medicine, for example, dishes made from ginger, sesame, and bone broth are often prescribed to help warm the body, prevent cold, and increase circulation. Rich, hearty foods fortify the mother and aid in her recovery.

The principle behind these foods is not just about physical nourishment but also restoring "balance" in the body. Traditional postpartum practices emphasize the importance of protecting the new mother's health by aligning her body with the natural rhythms of healing.

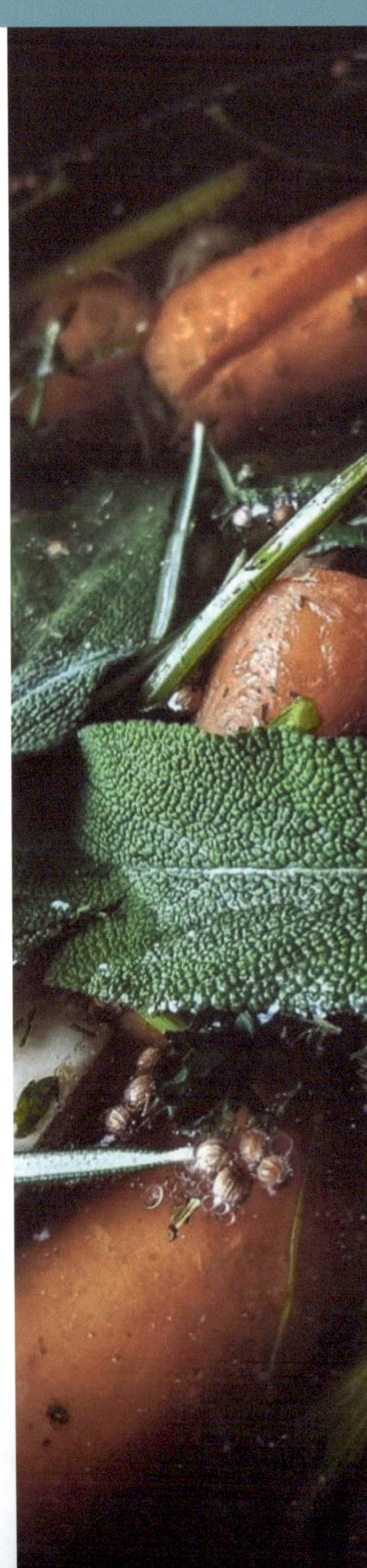

Rest and Support: Central to traditional postpartum practices is rest—both physical and mental. In many societies, the new mother is encouraged to remain in bed or at home, resting and focusing solely on recovery and bonding with her newborn. This is a radical contrast to western society's tendency to encourage early participation in normal activities. In these traditions, rest is not seen as indulgent or lazy or unnecessary, but as essential to the healing process.

Extended family members or close friends should be involved in helping with household duties, cooking, and child care, allowing the new mother to focus entirely on her own well-being and the initial bonding experience with her baby. The emotional support from family members is another cornerstone of traditional postpartum care. Postpartum depression, "baby blues" and other postpartum hormone imbalances can affect many new mothers, and these traditions often acknowledge the importance of mental and emotional health. The presence of close family members or a supportive community network is a solution to isolation, providing the new mother with a nurturing environment in which she feels both cared for and cherished.

Traditional Practices from Around the World:
• The "Confinement" Period in China: As mentioned, many Chinese women observe a month-long period of rest known as "zuo yuezi," or "sitting the month." During this time, mothers avoid cold foods and drinks, stay indoors, and limit their physical activities. The focus is on nurturing the mother through a combination of dietary practices, warmth, and rest.

• The "Cuarentena" in Latin America: In many Latin American cultures, the cuarentena is a 40-day period where the new mother is kept at home and supported by her family. It is a time for recuperation and reflection. Traditional foods such as "tamales" and "caldos" are made to ensure the mother receives essential nutrients.

• The "Quarantine" in Indonesia: In Indonesia, a common postpartum practice involves "traditional jamu," a herbal medicine made from turmeric, ginger, and other local plants. These are believed to aid in postpartum recovery, promote healing, and balance the body's energy.

• The "Sitz Bath" in Europe: In parts of Europe, new mothers often take warm herbal baths to soothe their bodies after childbirth. These baths are made from a blend of herbs like lavender, calendula, and chamomile, which are known for their calming, healing properties.

Fostering a Strong Bond with Baby: At its core, traditional postpartum care focuses not just on the physical recovery of the mother but also the nurturing of the bond between mother and baby. Whether through "skin-to-skin" practices, co-sleeping, or constant caregiving, these traditions recognize the deep emotional needs of both mother and child during this period. The first few months are often seen as a time to focus entirely on the infant's needs, promoting breastfeeding, close contact, and attachment. In many cultures, the support of extended family and community during this time allows the mother to fully engage with her newborn without feeling overwhelmed. This communal approach also reinforces the idea that motherhood is not a solitary endeavor but one that is shared and supported by a community of loving individuals.

Experiencing a slow traditional postpartum period offers invaluable space for deep healing and bonding as a family. This rest, nourishment, and postpartum support allows mothers to renew and establish deep connections with their newborns in a peaceful, nurturing environment. By honoring this sacred time, new mothers can experience a more balanced recovery, giving long-term well-being and a deeper sense of resilience as they step into motherhood with both care and confidence.

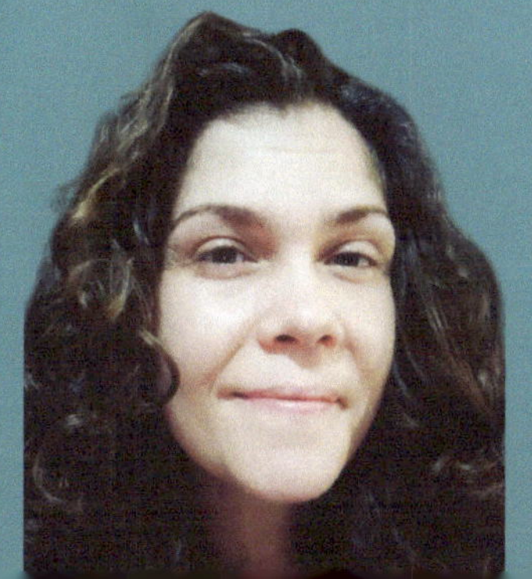

Stephenie Ignacio, *The Nourished Mother*
Postpartum Doula and Postpartum Nutrition Counselor.
@The Nourished Mother on Facebook
Based in Portland, Oregon

From Fear to Fierce:
An Evolution of Birthing Experiences

By Nicole Harlot

"No, I don't want a mirror,
I don't want to see anything that is going on down there.
I said to my doula as she was going over options for my first birth.

I was terrified of the scene. I was so fearful of the pain.
I couldn't fathom the entire experience.

Then, I did it. I birthed my first baby boy.
Empowered and Supported in a hospital.

My body knew it's potential all along.

My second boy came, my eyes opened wide.
I did it, again- this time on my terms.
Source had a greater plan and mission for me.

Then two bedroom babies were birthed into our family.

One very quick dance with my beautiful daughter-
celebrated in sisterhood in my home.

Then a challenging entrance where, still- there was no mirror,
but my hands were who caught my baby boy.

My fear turned to a fierce mama who births with a roar and
knows just how powerful her body, mind and spirit truly are.

This feeling I hope that all women could experience.

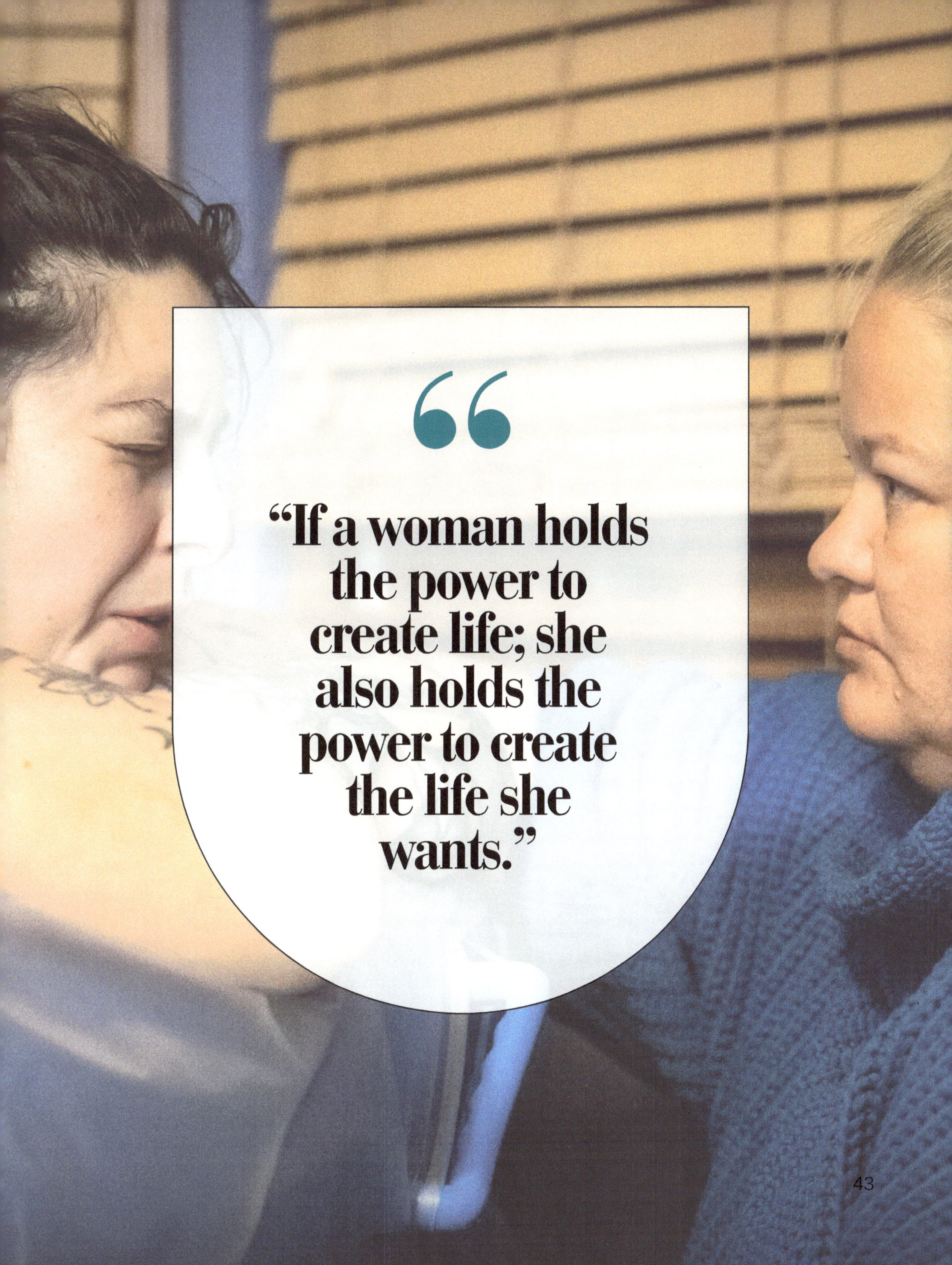
"If a woman holds the power to create life; she also holds the power to create the life she wants."

THANK YOU!

From the bottom of my heart & womb, I am so grateful for every women, mother and supporter that is reading this magazine, has contributed to this magazine in some way, and for anyone sharing it!

The concept, implementation and distribution is not easy along with many other projects in the works but I am so excited for it to be live and for YOU to get even just one thing from these words.

I am hopeful that as the Perinatal Resource Collaborative grows and expands we will be able to offer issues more frequently but for now as the seasons are upon up, we will birth and deliver a new collection of resources, stories, and articles to share.

This is such a labor of love and a passion of mine- and I am thrilled to bring it to life.

Please provide any feedback and share with others if it has helped you in anyway!

If you are reading the print version of this in an office or place of business- be sure to scan the code below to subscribe to the digital version for free!

Nicole Harlet

xo ♡